Arrest the Silent Killer

Surviving Ovarian Cancer:
a guide and memoir

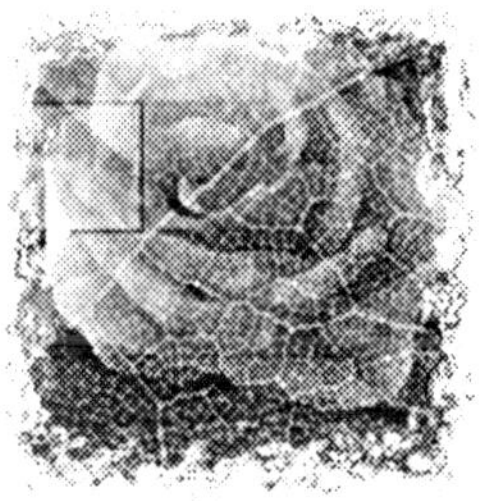

Marion Seferth

About the Author

Marion Seferth grew up and was educated in suburban Melbourne before training as a nurse in the early '60s. She married soon after graduating and settled in a semi-

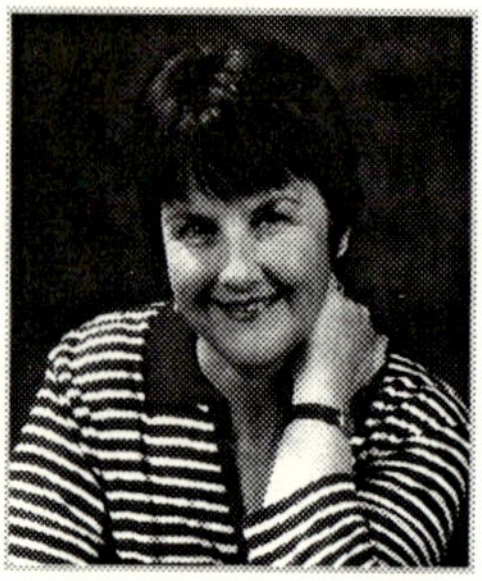

rural area. Suburbia caught up with them, so she and her husband and two children moved to a hobby farm in the Yarra Valley, where she wrote about her experiences there for numerous magazines and local newspapers. They separated when the children were teenagers, and she later remarried and settled in Healesville, where she wrote a series of children's books. She moved to Northeast Victoria after her second marriage ended, where she wrote this book in the idyllic farm setting of El Dorado, close to her beloved grandsons.

Published in Australia by
Temple House Pty Ltd,
T/A Sid Harta Publishers
ACN 092 197 192
Hartwell, Victoria

Telephone: 61 3 9560 9920
Facsimile: 61 3 9545 1742
E-mail: author@sidharta.com.au

First published in Australia 2004

Cover design, typesetting: Chameleon Print Design

Photograph of Marion Seferth
by Occasion Studios, Wangaratta.

National Library of Australia Cataloguing-in-Publication entry:
Seferth, Marion
Arrest the Silent Killer
ISBN: 1-877059-64-1
pp260

Printed by Wordsworth Books.
Typeset in Book Antiqua

ii

Marion Seferth has been very generous in allowing us to read about her personal journey with ovarian cancer. Through her story we are made aware of how important the support of family and close friends is during a time of crisis. Each person experiences cancer in a different way and makes personal choices regarding treatment and ways of keeping as healthy as possible. For others experiencing a similar disease, it is so important to be able to know that they are not alone in their feelings and experiences. I was especially impressed with the section regarding palliative care. Palliative care is an excellent way of providing pain and symptom control at any point in one's cancer journey yet all too often it is perceived as only being for the last weeks of life. I wish Marion good health and happiness for the future and thank her for letting us accompany her on her journey. For cancer information and support the Cancer Helpline 13 11 20 is a valuable resource.

Doreen Akkerman, Director, Cancer Information and Support Service, The Cancer Council Victoria

Preface

This is a book about hope.

Hope that the label of 'The Silent Killer', presently attached to ovarian cancer, will fade into mythology as doctors become more aware of, and alert to, the early signs and symptoms.

Hope that medical technology will facilitate earlier diagnosis.

Hope that gene research will enable women to be more aware of their vulnerability.

Hope that scientific research will reveal drugs that can cure this presently incurable disease, once it has spread.

It is the story of my personal encounter and journey with advanced ovarian cancer. I want to share my experiences, both good and bad, but more importantly to instill in the hearts and minds of all, that we each have a part to play in our own destiny. For me, fighting this insidious disease is about holistic medicine; exploring and treating body, mind and spirit. It is a partnership between patient, medical science and natural therapies.

My earnest belief is in the power of the mind to heal, which I feel I have proved to myself through my personal experience.

This book is also dedicated to the thousands of women who have suffered and died from ovarian cancer and its complications, some of whom I count among my dearest friends, and to the families and friends who have watched in despair and been left bereft.

v

Most importantly, it is for my daughter Katrina who has supported me throughout my long and arduous journey. My greatest wish is to help to eradicate any uncertainty she might have about her own future.

ACKNOWLEDGEMENTS

I wish to take this opportunity to offer my sincere thanks to the following people:

Katrina, for the idea of this book and for encouragement and memory jogging.

To Margrit and my fellow students in the class of 2002 at TAFE, Wangaratta for guidance and feedback.

To Pauline and Joan for patient early proof reading and suggestions.

To Jenny, Les and Debbie, my doctors, for their information and advice, and for verifying the medical information.

To my wonderful oncology nurses for keeping me going and checking over Appendix 5.

To OVCA Australia, and especially Director Simon Lee and his late wife who set up the web site, for support, encouragement and resources.

To Bob for setting up my computer, and Greg and Katrina for paper.

To Kerry at Sid Harta for accepting my manuscript, and my editor Jackie for her work on the final edit.

To all my family and friends for their love, support and encouragement.

Dedication

For:

my family, friends and guardian angels,
in this life, and the next.

Contents

CHAPTER 1

Just take a look - the pursuit of diagnosis

My Story

"It's not fair! Why did this have to happen to me? All I've ever wanted in life was love and harmony, and now my life is one of pain and tension. Where did I go wrong? How can I fix it?"

These were the thoughts tearing through my mind and heart, as I lay in pain, unable to sleep. I could feel a hard lump in my abdomen where a lump shouldn't be, and its presence terrified me. Why couldn't I get any answers, any action? Why, why, why?

This was the beginning of my journey with ovarian cancer. I am just one of thousands of women with similar stories.

In telling my story I'm tempted to stick to dates and symptoms, tests and outcomes, as this is all recorded as it happened in my daily journal. But this would only be telling half the story. I'm not just a body this disease happened to, I'm a wife, daughter, mother, grandmother, workmate, friend, and all these relationships are an integral part of who I am and how I live my life.

At the time my body was showing signs of disease, I was living in the semi-rural town of Healesville, in the Yarra Valley of central Victoria. The most dominant factor in my life was the relationship with my second husband,

Ted. When I resigned from nursing in 1992 following my third severe back injury, Ted developed manic depression or bipolar disorder, as it is now known. What's in a name – it's the same debilitating disease. It is described medically as being 'characterized by manic episodes, which refer to a period dominated by an elevated, expansive and irritable mood that is severe enough to impair occupational and social function. Patients with bipolar disorder usually also experience major depressive episodes.' This was descriptive of Ted's behavior. Research shows that this illness may be accelerated by a loss, in Ted's case, his physical ability to work due to advanced lung disease. Mental illness can be cruel, changing personalities and destroying relationships. If only Ted had acknowledged he had a problem and accepted the medical and psychological help offered, things might have turned out differently – but then, perhaps they weren't meant to.

Also, during the summer of '96/97 — one of the hottest on record — I had some added distractions: my elderly mother who lived over the road from us, was going through a series of minor and one major operation for numerous skin cancers, we had a very large garden to maintain, which was mainly my responsibility, and I also worked as a pharmacy assistant one week in two.

My son Greg, and daughter-in-law Jane, lived not too far away in suburban Melbourne. But my daughter Katrina, her partner Rob, and my grandson Thomas, were over 200kms away on a farm at Byawatha, on the outskirts of Wangaratta in Northeast Victoria. I greatly missed regular close contact with them.

Earliest signs

Tuesday 5th November 1996. Melbourne Cup Day, the day a Nation stops for a horse race.

I awoke early with acute pain over the area of my left ovary, which had persisted since the previous Saturday. Ever since I'd had an emergency Caesarian Section in 1970 for the birth of my second and last child, I had been aware of when I ovulated, characterised by some discomfort on either my right or left side at that time in my cycle. The discomfort had never been sufficient to complain to the doctor about until now. But this time I was worried.

As this was a public holiday a doctor was not on duty, so I took some aspirin and persevered. As always, I retreated to the garden to forget my worries, and happily filled the day weeding, mulching, and planting vegetable seeds. By the time the Cup was run I felt much better, and finished the day by walking Waminda my beloved, old German Shepherd dog. I had 'inherited' Waminda from my daughter when she had left home to live on a farm. Still, I decided to have a medical check up.

I rang for a doctor's appointment the following morning before going to work. My GP's opinion after examining me was that I had a larger than usual ovarian cyst. An ultrasound was ordered for the Friday to confirm his diagnosis, and an appointment to see him the following Tuesday to discuss the result was made.

The pain persisted overnight Thursday, but settled down after breakfast, enabling me to keep myself busy outside until it was time for the ultrasound late that afternoon. The radiographer's opinion was that it looked like a large cyst plus 'something else' - the official results would be available by lunchtime the following day. The pain returned that evening.

After receiving the report, my GP rang me and suggested I make an appointment with a gynaecologist, but the earliest appointment I could get was in February!

My daughter Katrina rang that evening to confirm she

would be coming down to visit over the weekend, which cheered me up.

Katrina, with eleven and a half months old Thomas, called in on Sunday on their way to visit her paternal grandmother, known as Granny, who was terminally ill. My son Greg and his wife Jane also visited with a trailer load of mulch for the garden, which had to be unloaded and spread. On their way home to Byawatha on Tuesday, Katrina and Thomas called in again - and so life went on with its day-to-day demands.

Sunday 17th November. Katrina rang to say Thomas was walking.

The following Friday, Ted and I were up early as we were going to Byawatha for Thomas's first birthday party, and a pre-arranged tandem parachute jump I was going to do at Nagambie. This was a gift from Katrina and Greg for my 50th birthday in May 1994. The weather had not been appropriate on previous attempts, so hopefully I would do it this trip. Ted tore a muscle in his chest while putting the trailer on the car, necessitating painkillers and a cup of tea to ease the pain, but we were still on the road by 8.30am, arriving at Katrina's three hours later.

After finalizing the party preparations, there was time for me to enjoy playing with Thomas. The party in the evening was a great success, but unfortunately for Ted, his persistent pain made it a strain for him. We stayed overnight in a cabin at a nearby caravan park.

The drive to Nagambie for my jump the next day entailed an early start. The weather was perfect, but we had to wait around until after lunch for the man who was to jump with me and record it on videotape.

Parachuting was a fantastic experience and over too soon. My first impression when we exited the plane was of how cold the air was we were rushing through, but then, we were over a mile high. After landing, the pilot commented that I hadn't seemed at all afraid. I said 'Of course not, this was something I wanted to do!' I have always had a great love of flying, and was well on my way to obtaining my Private Pilot's License, until a back injury in my early 30's caused whilst nursing, put an end to the income that was funding the lessons. For me, the parachute jump was just a natural extension of that love.

On arriving back at the farm, the family watched the video and was suitably impressed!

Before departing the following day, Thomas held his arms out to me to be picked up. This was a first, and made me very happy.

Ted was still in a lot of discomfort, so I made a doctor's appointment for him when we got home. He had been fairly emotionally stable for the past four months, so it came as a shock when he started performing, accusing me of not caring about his pain and of flirting with men at the party. (If I commented about the weather to a man it constituted flirting in Ted's eyes). He forbade me to go to Byawatha alone in the future and raved on and on, his imagination in full flight. This was all typical of earlier behavior, and I could stand it no longer. For the first time in our married life I slept (or tried to), in the spare room, which made him even angrier and he stomped around the house for hours.

The next day I kept out of Ted's way by going over to Mum's and doing some gardening for her, and later took her shopping. By the following day, Ted and I were able to talk and resolve issues sufficiently to get on with day-to-day life, though Ted sank into depression for the next few days.

This may all sound a bit dramatic, but I had endured

living with my husband's unreasonable moods and outbursts before, and dreaded going through all the drunken ravings, smashing of things and suicide threats again. Usually performed just as we were sitting down to a meal, or in the middle of the night, these incidents made me emotionally fragile. Ted at this stage was nothing like the person I knew and loved during the first five years of our relationship and marriage.

We met when my first marriage was in its death throes, and his was at a turning point. I fulfilled a long held desire to learn ballroom dancing, and Ted was one of the teachers. He was a talented dancer and excellent teacher, and when he partnered me, he led so well I felt I could dance far better than I actually could; I'll never forget our first waltz together, and our last many years later.

I was reluctant to start another relationship and put off his advances for many months, but once my separation was finalized and I had a home of my own, we started seeing each other out of class time, and despite him being eighteen years older than me, we fell deeply in love.

Our families were not as enchanted with the relationship as we were, but after we bought our own home together and got married, things settled down, though Mum was never comfortable with Ted.

We did some wonderful trips together - Western Australia, Tasmania, and New Zealand - and we formed a great team creating our beautiful garden.

What happened? Ted had smoked since an early age, and continued to do so all his working life. Combined with his asthma, he had developed severe emphysema, and his lungs and breathing had deteriorated to the stage that he was no longer able to dance, teach dancing, or to help maintain the garden that was on a steeply sloping site.

As long as Ted felt in charge and in control he was fine, but without his physical and creative outlets he felt lost and inadequate. He wasn't able to re-channel his energies and adapt to his limitations, but dwelt on the negative aspects of what he wanted to do but was no longer physically capable of doing. On top of that, Ted developed cataracts in both eyes which limited even more the few things he did that gave him pleasure, such as building and mending things in his workshop, and doing crossword puzzles. And so the frustration and boredom played havoc with his mind and his life became a nightmare to him. My ability to still do what ever I wanted must have been an added thorn in his side, so he attacked me in frustration – this is how I saw and understood the situation.

Yet I had loved Ted so much, with a passion I didn't even imagine I possessed, and when we danced together we were in such perfect unity, people stopped dancing to watch us. Our hours in the garden together were harmonious and fulfilling – a great team. After a hard day's work, we loved to relax with a barbecue, and contemplate with satisfaction the results of our labor.

It is these happy times I wanted to remember.

Action

Tuesday 3rd December. Stomach pains disturbed my sleep, lodging over my left ovary by morning. I rang John (my boss) to say I wouldn't be in to work, and then went back to bed until I could see my GP later that day.

The doctor could feel the ovarian cyst this time, so he ordered another ultrasound, which I had soon after. The cyst had grown to 18cm across. I went straight back to the GP, who rang the nearest hospital and arranged for me to be admitted that night. I arrived in casualty at 9pm where I was given an injection to ease the pain, and was eventually admitted to a ward.

Sleep evaded me, but the pain eased and I passed the next day reading and taking phone calls from the family. Katrina already had enough worries as Rob was sick and Granny had deteriorated. Following blood tests, an ECG, and a visit from the anaesthetist, I was wheeled off to theatre where the surgeon drained the cyst and performed a curette.

The ward's resident doctor came around early the next morning and said I could go home, with instructions to return to the outpatients department six weeks later to discuss removal of my left fallopian tube. I never actually spoke to the surgeon, and don't know to this day if it was a man or a woman!

A huge bunch of flowers from my work colleagues was awaiting me when I arrived home, and Mum brought over heaps of food for tea. Katrina rang later to say she would be down for the weekend.

I slept well that night, but was still pretty sore, so I rested and read for most of the following day. Ted gave me my Christmas present early, a cordless phone, which was charged and ready for me to use by my chair in the lounge. It came in very handy. Katrina rang in the late afternoon to say Granny had died earlier that day.

Greg and Jane arrived about 4pm on Saturday, and Katrina and Thomas half an hour later. They were all laden with food, which we enjoyed later as a family feast. Thomas was walking all the time by now, and he was very sociable – such a joy. I was feeling better just having my family around me.

Katrina and I enjoyed the rest of her stay together, during which she also spent time with Mum and did some domestic chores for me. A visit from my life-long friend, Margot, was another pleasant diversion. Ted hibernated in his workshop and was barely civil during this time.

With their departure, Ted and I went shopping to replenish supplies. I was rather sore and tired when I got home and depressed about Ted's behavior, and the departure of my family.

The dark mood was still with me the following morning and I had a big cry while Ted was outside, which helped ease my tension. I had an appointment with my GP later on that Tuesday. He told me about the letter he had received from the surgeon who had drained the cyst, commenting that it wasn't so much the size of the cyst, but the size of the ovary that was the problem. My GP then wrote a letter to the gynaecologist I was to see in February, updating all that had occurred.

I returned to work on the 13th and life went on as usual, with pre-Christmas preparations, garden maintenance, housework and my job keeping me busy. Ted remained moody.

Monday 16th December. I worked all day, and as we were one assistant short, I stayed on until 6pm. When I arrived home, Ted said he wanted to talk. He then launched into a list of all the things some of my family members had ever (supposedly) done to upset him, and expected me to just listen and not react. I told him I was sick of his endless criticism, and poured myself a drink of brandy and dry ginger, an unusual event, and refused to cook tea. Ted wouldn't allow me to watch TV, so I retired to the bedroom and cried. He tried intervening, but I told him to leave me alone. I didn't know when he'd sleep or what would happen next, and was past caring.

I had a terrible night, and developed a thumping headache and a sore throat before taking some medication and a hot drink around 3am. I finally got a little sleep, but I couldn't bring myself to speak to Ted before going to work.

The following day the air had cleared sufficiently to talk a few things out.

Christmas Day dawned, and we were up early, ready for a wonderful family day. The house and Christmas tree were looking very festive, and I had gone to a lot of trouble setting the table and arranging flowers. Seeing Thomas's delight and excitement was the best part, and I was able to forget my worries as we all enjoyed ourselves, four generations of my little family together around the table. On Boxing Day, all Ted's family came and we repeated the celebrations.

I love Christmas. Childhood Christmases were full of excited anticipation and wishes come true. There was always a Christmas tree; a branch from the huge pines on my parent's block in the then rural suburb of Mooroolbark.

Early post-war, the tree was decorated with only Christmas cards and cotton wool, then tinsel and colored glass balls were introduced. To us, it was always beautiful. We would leave our pillowcase 'stockings' near the tree, and would creep out at first light to see what Father Christmas had brought for us. My much longed for bride doll is my fondest memory.

For many years our grandparents joined us at midday for a traditional roast dinner, with Christmas pudding completing the meal. Mum always made sure we each had money hidden in our slice, a threepence or sixpence. One year, I completed my serve without finding the money and was heart-broken. Knowing that a threepenny bit had been inserted, Mum was in a dilemma. I expect I was recompensed, I don't really remember, but Dad always said I was worth threepence after that.

My worst Christmas was the one following my first marriage. We had invited my in-laws for lunch, and I was out to impress. I got up early and roasted a duck, and put it on the kitchen bench covered with a tea towel while we went to church. It was a hot day with a strong North wind, and the sliding wire door was blown open sufficiently to allow a blow fly to enter. It found my duck, and when we got home the maggots were having a feast. It was the end of the world for me, and I was inconsolable. My husband rang his parents and explained the situation, and they detoured for miles on their trip to our place to buy a ready-cooked chicken; total humiliation for me.

Early in my married life, I found a recipe for a rich, fruity plum pudding that was absolutely delicious, and from that year to this I have made that pudding, usually in October to give it time to mature. Even if we can't be together as a family on Christmas day, we eat it together when we celebrate the Season.

When we had our own children, the magic of Christmas returned. Watching the delight and surprise on our children's faces when Father Christmas had brought just what they wanted is one of the most joyous and rewarding parts of parenthood. My most precious possession is a tape recording of my children singing carols.

Grandchildren have brought the magic back yet again. Trees are more elegantly dressed these days, but mine contains decorations made by my children, and souvenirs of happy occasions and friendships. Some are looking their age, as I am, but for me, Christmas is about memories. Katrina also loves Christmas, and I know she will carry on the family traditions, and encourage her children to do so too.

Tests, and more tests

As the first day of 1997 dawned, I wondered what it would bring. Would Ted, Mum and Wim survive the year? Would our marriage?

The hot, dry summer continued, with seemingly endless garden watering. During the first week of the New Year, we recorded the hottest night for five years.

Friday 10th January started with a sleepless night of pain and worry, which made me decide to bring my appointment with the gynaecologist forward a week to late January.

The weekend was spent endlessly moving hoses and hand watering pots. I was still bleeding heavily when I menstruated, and experiencing a lot of back pain - which I had been free of for several years - and getting rather depressed about it all. I made an appointment with the osteopath for Monday, to see if he could give me some relief. He was of the opinion that my back had probably been injured while under anaesthetic. This I could well imagine, having worked in theatre and seen the unnatural postures unconscious patients are put in. With the help of his 'magic' hands, the pain started easing in a few days.

20th January was 42C. I checked that Mum was keeping cool and having plenty to drink, and I kept poor old Wim wet all day to cool her off.

It was still very hot on the day I had to attend my out patients appointment. My surgeon was not available. I was seen by a young Asian resident without enough English to communicate effectively, which made me feel my appointment was a waste of time. I asked for a letter to take to my own gynaecologist, hoping to get the whole business resolved.

Monday 27th January. At last the day dawned that I was to see my own gynaecologist and hopefully get some personal attention and resolution. He wrote down my medical history and read the letters from my GP and the hospital, before giving me a thorough physical examination. He said he was not sure what the lump was, and wanted another ultrasound done before making a decision. I was disappointed at the delay, and my mood matched the storm that was brewing as we drove home. Waminda was terrified of thunderstorms, and ran off in terror at the first clap of thunder before I had the chance to secure her. After the storm had passed, I walked for miles calling her but to no avail. She finally turned up many hours later soaking wet and exhausted.

The following Thursday I went for the ultrasound, and it was found that the cyst had filled again. When I saw the gynaecologist the following day, he booked me in at the local hospital for the 9th of April, to have my uterus and left ovary removed. He was still not totally convinced that the lump was all to do with my ovary, and wanted me to have a colonoscopy before the operation. The inference that my bowel might be involved upset me, as my worst nightmare had always been the occurrence of bowel cancer, with a resulting colostomy and accompanying bag.

I hardly slept that night, and not just because it was hot and humid. I was worried and in pain, aching all over with tension, and my back was agony. Ted was withdrawn and moody, and Mum was struggling to cope with the heat and humidity; I felt so alone and unhappy.

I spent the weekend alternately resting while the pain was at its worst, and pottering around doing domestic chores while the analgesics were having affect.

February 3rd. When I saw my GP to arrange for the colonoscopy, he said I wouldn't be able to get an appointment as a public patient for months, long after the date for the operation. He examined me and decided a barium enema would serve the same purpose, and made an appointment for me to have it done the following day, Tuesday.

My day started at 5am with the first of many trips to the toilet as the bowel prep medication took affect. The barium enema was uncomfortable but routine, and everyone was very kind. Once home, I rested my aching back between numerous trips to the toilet to evacuate the barium.

The following day I started menstruating, with the heavy bleeding I had been experiencing over the last few months, due, I was told, to some small fibroids in my uterus.

It was at about this time I was lent a book, entitled *What your Doctor May Not Tell You About Menopause – the breakthrough book on natural progesterone*, by John R. Lee M.D. I read it thoroughly and it made a lot of sense to me. Two facts particularly interested me.

1. 'An alternative treatment for ovarian cysts is natural progesterone. The signaling mechanism that shuts off ovulation in one ovary each cycle is the production of progesterone in the other. If sufficient natural progesterone is supplemented prior to ovulation, LH levels are inhibited and both ovaries think the other has ovulated, so regular ovulation does not occur. Therefore, adding natural progesterone from day 10 – 26 of the cycle suppresses LH and its luteinizing effects. Thus the ovarian cyst will not be stimulated and, in the passage of one or two such monthly cycles, will very likely shrink and disappear without further treatment.'
2. 'Fibroids are one of the most common reasons that women in their 30s and 40s have a hysterectomy. Here again, natural progesterone offers a better

alternative. Fibroid tumors are a product of oestrogen dominance. Oestrogen stimulates their growth, and lack of oestrogen causes them to atrophy (shrink). As (women) approach the decade before menopause they are producing much less progesterone than expected, but still producing normal oestrogen. When sufficient progesterone is replaced, fibroid tumors no longer grow in size (they generally decrease in size), and can be kept from growing until menopause, after which they will atrophy. This is the effect of reverting oestrogen dominance.'

I decided to purchase some natural progesterone cream and try it out. When I saw my GP for the result of the barium enema, which showed a normal bowel, I told him of my plan.

When I ovulated in early February, pain prevented me attending work for three days. I commenced applying the progesterone cream to my forearms before retiring on the 13th of February, and used it nightly until the 25th.

When I would normally have ovulated in early March, I was pain-free, so I guessed the natural progesterone cream was working. Hooray!

Tuesday 11th March. I went to see my GP to get a form to have another ultrasound before seeing the gynaecologist again. We discussed the effect the cream was having, and his opinion was that a hysterectomy was unnecessary, as I was close to menopause when the fibroids would no longer be a problem. When I saw my osteopath a couple of days later, he felt the lump in my lower abdomen and suggested I ask for a laparoscopic examination to ascertain its true nature before having any radical surgery; it certainly made sense to me. Trying to convince a doctor to do such a procedure was to be another matter. All they seemed to be interested in doing was sending me off for more tests.

The ultrasound showed no sign of the cyst, and the extensive work the osteopath had done on my back had relieved the pain to a great extent.

Ted and I had another trip to see Katrina a week later, where I spent some special time with Thomas. As usual, Ted was difficult and moody after we got home, and even though I tried to detach myself from his outbursts, it was upsetting, but he settled down after a few days.

Friday 21st March. I went to see my GP for the official report on the ultrasound. It was reported as 'normal'. He examined me once more and could still feel the lump, so now he too thought it might be on my bowel and ordered a colonoscopy. My heart sank. No sooner did I think I had solved my problem and could get on with my life, than I was knocked down again with more doubts. All the uncertainty and delay upset me to the point that I couldn't eat, and having to seek urgent medical treatment for Mum's bronchitis over the weekend didn't help.

Monday 24th March was the appointment day with my gynaecologist. After reading the ultrasound report and examining me, he now considered the lump had nothing to do with my ovary, and cancelled my operation, suggesting I saw a general surgeon. I obtained the required referral from my GP the next day, and rang for an appointment for the following Tuesday.

Katrina rang over the weekend to say Rob had glandular fever and she had a sore throat. How I wished everything was normal and I could have been there to help out.

April started with a crisp morning (1.6°C) then developed into a lovely sunny day. The summer had been exhausting – February that year had been the hottest on record so far this century, in Victoria, with no rain. Thank goodness Mum had decided to have air conditioning installed earlier that month. I took Mum shopping in the morning, then after lunch Ted and I went shopping and visited his elder daughter Anne before my appointment with the surgeon. After physically examining me, he was very vague, and said I needed to have a colonoscopy before he could come to any definite conclusion, so his receptionist tried to get an earlier date than the one I already had.

The next few days saw me back in the usual routine of work and domestic duties. Rain brought the endless watering to an end - thank goodness - but Ted's moods continued to swing; the weather seemed to be a major influence.

I received a letter from the surgeon's rooms with a date in June for my colonoscopy. That seemed forever away, and the lack of action when I was clearly unwell was getting me down. I had gone from a fit and healthy woman six months previously, to one with a palpable lump increasing in size in my lower abdomen, increased heavy bleeding, a distended abdomen, fatigue, loss of appetite, weight loss, and all the medical profession did was to order more tests! Why couldn't someone have just taken a look?

After stewing this over, I rang the surgeon's receptionist and asked how much it would cost to have the colonoscopy done as a private patient.

The cost was exorbitant, but on a pension card (which I had as the wife of an aged pensioner), I could have it done at a reduced cost at a private hospital the following Thursday. This fitted in well with our planned trip to Byawatha earlier that week. I arranged to swap working days with one of my colleagues, and felt more in control of the situation.

The Friday before our scheduled trip, I posted all the paper work required to the Private Hospital and purchased the medication required as bowel preparation prior to the procedure, and started packing.

We travelled up to Byawatha on the Saturday, arriving in time for lunch. The afternoon was spent helping to collect firewood, which entailed driving out to one of the paddocks in the ute, where Rob used the chain saw to cut fallen trees into useable lengths. Katrina then split those she could, and Ted and I (mostly me) loaded the prepared wood into the ute. I have always loved our autumn wood gathering, and feel 'rich' when I see a good stack of wood ready for the winter. They have a combustion stove in the kitchen and a combustion heater in the lounge, so a lot of wood is required. We had a lovely dinner with them, and then went to our usual cabin in the caravan park for the night.

We didn't arrive back at Katrina's until mid morning and found they had already gone out for more wood. We relaxed on the verandah - always a very pleasant experience - until they arrived home, then we helped unload and stack the wood. Thomas and I were getting on very well, and he kept telling everyone that I was Grandma ('Ma Ma'), which gave me a warm glow.

Katrina and I gardened together in the afternoon while Ted listened to the football; he was a keen Hawthorn supporter. In the evening, Rob took Katrina out for dinner as a birthday treat, and we stayed to mind Thomas. This was the first time Thomas had been left with anyone but his parents, so it was a big step for all concerned, but everything went well.

We celebrated Katrina's birthday the following evening with a delicious meal cooked by Rob. His parents joined us, and it culminated in the cutting of the birthday cake, Thomas helping with the candle blowing of course.

Ted and I returned home the following day.

From midday, Wednesday, I had to start my bowel prep, and then spent a large amount of the evening and night on the toilet, very uncomfortable, as my back was painful after the wood gathering.

Thursday 17th April was colonoscopy day, and as fasting is required prior to this procedure, I was unable to take analgesics to relieve the severe sciatic pain I was experiencing. Hospital admission occurred at 11.30am, and Ted was told to return three hours later to take me home. What a joke: I was barely conscious by then and acute abdominal pain caused me to retch every time I moved, so the nurse gave me some injections. I was finally discharged at 5.30pm, but vomited upon arriving home, and went to bed. After getting rid of all the air they had pumped into my intestines during the procedure I felt a lot better.

As my sciatica was still very painful the next day, I lay down as much as possible. Ted's back was also troublesome, so he joined me and we just arose to eat and drink, which resulted in pain relief for us both by evening. On ringing the surgeon's rooms for the result of the colonoscopy, I was informed it was nothing serious, and was given an appointment for the following Tuesday.

I was back at work on Monday, and struggled through the day in pain. Ted was a little better thank goodness, but Mum had been to see her GP that day and been informed that the second lesion he had removed from her face was malignant, so more would have to be removed.

He also removed yet another skin cancer from her leg, making it an upsetting and painful day for her. Sleep was a welcome escape that night.

Tuesday 22nd April. At 12.30am, I awoke with severe pain in my abdomen and shoulder, which finally settled down after a couple of hours. I worked that morning, came home for lunch, and then rested until 4.30 when Ted drove me to see the surgeon again.

The surgeon was satisfied that my bowel appeared normal for a person my age, and considered the lump to be my uterus and fibroids, which would settle with menopause and need no treatment. I was happy to agree. I mentioned the new pain I had developed in the lower left-hand side of my abdomen, but he dismissed it lightly without examining me further. Now, I thought, I just have to fix my back and get on with my life. The good news was spread around the family that evening, and I made an appointment with the osteopath for Thursday.

The osteopath worked on my back for 3/4hr. He said it would hurt for 48hrs then become a lot better. He was certainly right about the pain. I hardly moved from my bed for the next two days. Relief slowly came and my back began to improve, but I had to cancel several outings.

By Sunday I was able to sit down for breakfast, but after a few domestic chores I had to go back to bed and lie down. To add insult to injury, I still had the annoying pain in my side, and a hyperactive bowel.

By Tuesday, the pain in my side was worse. My GP's opinion was that I had a bowel infection, probably from the colonoscopy, necessitating a course of antibiotics. He wanted a CT scan done when the infection cleared. I rested all afternoon, feeling rather depressed; would life ever be normal and pain-free again, I wondered? Mum came over with a lemon delicious dessert, my favorite, and I enjoyed some of that for tea.

On Wednesday, I had a sleepless night in severe pain. I rang my GP in the morning requesting a prescription for a stronger analgesic, and a certificate for Thursday to Saturday off work. Ted did the run to the surgery and work, and I was able to get up and potter around a bit when the tablets took affect.

I was feeling a lot better by the next day and could eat a reasonable amount, and only needed analgesics at bedtime. I had lost weight by then and was under 50kg, my usual weight being about 52kg.

By the weekend, the pain in my side and back had eased

sufficiently for us to visit Greg and Jane and deliver her belated birthday gift, a wooden wheelbarrow Ted had built. I supervised them setting it up with soil and plants and it looked great. We returned after lunch and I was glad to rest, as my abdomen was tender again.

Sunday 4th May. I awoke in severe pain in the early hours of the morning. Analgesics eventually eased the pain sufficiently for me to get a little more sleep (I felt like a mobile pharmacy). I saw a GP - not my usual one - later that morning, and he was appalled that I didn't have a positive diagnosis after all this time and tests. He insisted I arrange to have a CT scan the following day, and gave me the required form. I spent the remainder of the day resting and in the depths of depression.

I obtained a mid morning appointment on the Tuesday for the scan, and was told to consume two bottles of liquid before hand, one Monday evening and another early Tuesday. I must have had the cleanest bowel 'this side of the black stump' with all the bowel prep I had taken in the preceding weeks!

The scan took over an hour. I rested between frequent trips to the toilet when I got home. The radiologist rang in the evening to say he wanted me to come back in the morning for another barium enema, as something was showing on the scan he'd checked. My stomach sank and I got the shakes. I pulled myself together and rang my GP for an explanation; he thought I had Crohn's disease, a chronic inflammation of the bowel, and very difficult to treat. He expected that I would need an exploratory operation to verify it. I was devastated but I didn't dare tell Ted all the details, as he was upset enough with all that was going on.

Since I'd been so unwell, Ted had been doing most of

the driving, and this was a big strain since his cataracts had enlarged, severely limiting his peripheral vision, and making night driving out of the question for him, as oncoming lights rendered him virtually blind.

Wednesday 7th May. What a hideous day. I woke with a headache after a restless night and we left early to attend radiology for the barium enema. They were short staffed and running behind time, so I was left to lie on the cold hard X-ray table for half an hour or so, not good for my back. I started to feel ill, shaking, sweating, and nauseated. They decided I was too ill to have the barium enema, and sent me to the nearest public hospital where the emergency staff called in the general surgeon I had consulted previously. He ordered an ultrasound, blood tests, and intravenous re-hydration. I was so dehydrated, the resident doctor had a lot of trouble locating a vein. I was wheeled off to X-ray where the technician conducted a very thorough vaginal ultrasound. When results came through, it was decided the problem with my bowel was a reaction to the antibiotic and that I had an abscess or tumor on my left ovary, which I needed to consult my gynecologist about! Just before being discharged (and still not fully hydrated), the resident ordered another blood test, which turned out to be a CA-125, the first one I'd ever had. Some hormone-based cancers, such as prostate and ovarian cancer, give off an enzyme called a marker, which can be detected in a blood test, in the case of ovarian cancer, a CA-125 or a CEA (inhibin), depending on the type of tumor. They are not 100% accurate, but to my knowledge, are the best available at the present time.

Why hadn't any of my other doctors thought of it earlier, much earlier?

I was still feeling well below par when I got home, and had two cups of tea before falling exhausted into bed.

Next morning I made porridge for breakfast, but everything was still going straight through me, so I took anti-diarrhoea medication and went back to bed. By lunchtime I was able to tolerate soup and toast, and I enjoyed the baked custard and stewed apple Mum brought over for tea. All this turmoil and stress had played havoc with Ted, and he was difficult and argumentative, which upset me further. A positive note saved the day: I had a story published in the Weekly Times newspaper, and won a prize.

My sciatica plagued me again on Friday morning, so I rested after breakfast. Dear Mum came over with a casserole for us, and luckily Ted had cheered up a bit and was civil to her. I had an appointment with my usual GP in the afternoon, and he was shocked to hear my tale of woe, and was as keen as I was to see an end to it all.

By the Saturday I was feeling much better; even my back had improved. I caught up on housework and had a lovely chat with Katrina on the phone. She was so bright and happy, despite a mouse plague; I didn't have the heart to tell her all the details of the past week. We made plans for her to come down for my birthday on the 16th of May.

Sunday 11th, Mother's Day. Greg and Jane arrived with a late breakfast of pancakes, one of my favorites. Greg washed up and then he Jane and myself went for a walk with Wim. When they left in the middle of the day, I went over and spent some time with Mum. In the evening, Ted and I saw the film *Evita* at the local cinema; she died of ovarian cancer, it was thought!

On Monday I picked a big bunch of roses from the garden and went for lunch with a close friend. Joan and I, along with Margot, had known each other at primary school, but had long since lost touch. We met again in '93 when I did VCE Psychology at the local community center; she was the tutor. We had since become very close, and she was the understanding ear that kept me going when Ted was at his worst. Thank goodness for dear Joan.

We chatted for five hours and I told her what had happened with my body, and that I had no idea what the future held, but just needed the whole business resolved one way or another. We hugged as we parted, and I went home feeling much calmer.

Tuesday 13th May, a date etched forever in my memory. I had an appointment with my gynaecologist in the morning to get the results of the CA-125. It was 1,116! He was so alarmed when he saw it, he wanted me to see the head of gynaecology and obstetrics at the hospital as soon as possible, and said he would arrange an appointment. Ted and I were just sitting down to lunch when I received the phone call with the appointment time of 3.30pm. I packed some basics in a bag 'just in case', and off we went. As soon as the doctor examined me, he arranged for me to be admitted for surgery first thing the next morning.

The end – and a new beginning

Ovarian Cancer; spread to my bowel and liver; total hysterectomy, bladder adhered to uterus; omentum removed – riddled with tumors; tumor on sigmoid colon – 12cm of bowel removed. (This was later described to me as Stage 3B, Grade 3, advanced ovarian cancer. (*See Appendix 1, 'What is Ovarian Cancer'*)

Twice the surgeon who had operated came to visit me to tell me this tale of gloom and doom. Racked with pain, the future looked so black I just wanted to die. I remember saying, "I want to die and be with my babies."

Between having Katrina and Greg, I had miscarried twice, each time at about 22 weeks. Those babies were so real to me, moving in my womb, and I lactated each time, making it even harder to bear. In those days you were told to go home and forget about it; no seeing the baby and time to grieve. I had carried that grief and loss all those years without conscious thought. In later years I tried to find out what had become of their bodies, but to no avail.

Friday 16th May. My 53rd birthday, the worst birthday of my life. Katrina brought Mum in to see me and she broke down and wept uncontrollably, much to her embarrassment. It was so hard for her - like re-living the past - as Dad had died of cancer at my age, and she and I had nursed him at home for as long as we could. The day before he died in hospital, Mum and my sister Brenda had a car accident on the way in to visit him and were unable to see him. I had visited Dad that day and found him unconscious and jaundiced. I kissed him and told him I loved him, feeling it would be goodbye. He died at six the next morning.

Everyone was so kind during my hospital stay. My room was overflowing with beautiful flowers and there was a constant stream of visitors, more than I could cope with in the first few days as I was so ill. Ted and Greg were at my bedside when I came out of theatre. Ted came every day for the first couple of weeks, but never offered to bring Mum, which I found incredible and hurtful. Because his cataracts made driving so stressful, he spent some time with his daughter Anne who lived close to the hospital. Ted asked Greg if he'd take Wim to his place as they had dogs of their own and an enclosed backyard. Wim's alternative was long, lonely days on the chain at home with no walks. She was thirteen years old by then and arthritic in the hindquarters, but still loved her daily walks, though they were now more like rambles. While at Greg's, Wim developed an infection and despite antibiotics, her condition deteriorated and her kidneys failed. Poor Greg had to make the decision whether to have her put down or not. When the decision was made he then had to tell me about it, and I was devastated; what else could go wrong?

My hospitalization was not a totally negative experience, of course. Among my numerous visitors were old friends I had not seen for many years, or only briefly, and we had some terrific conversations. Brenda lent me her Walkman, which filled my sleepless nights and helped me relax. Her partner Kaye, gave me Ian Gawler's book '*You Can Conquer Cancer*', which filled me with hope and enabled me to face the future more positively. An old friend, Bob brought in some early primary school readers he'd found at a market, and read me excerpts such as *The Hobyahs*.

"Through the blue gums came the hobyahs, run, run, running.

Skip, skip, skipping on the ends of their toes ran the hobyahs."

This triggered much mirth and reminiscences. He also brought in his daughter, Rebecca, my goddaughter, whom I hadn't seen since she was a child. She had her two children with her, and as Katrina and Thomas were visiting at the same time, it was a great reunion.

Another unexpected visitor was the gynaecologist I had consulted after I had the cyst drained. He came in to apologize for not investigating the possibility of ovarian cancer.

Ted gave up visiting me – the strain of driving had become too much - and I had to admit I was relieved. A very kindly social worker visited me in hospital, and I unburdened myself to her about my relationship with Ted over the last few years. I guess talking helped clarify the situation in my mind, and the sense of relief when Ted stopped visiting made me realize I had to make a choice; my marriage or my life. I chose life without him, and it was the greatest gift I have ever given myself.

CHAPTER 2
The fight for survival

Action at last, but too late

I had been left with so many unanswered questions. Why didn't the surgeon who drained the cyst in December '96 do a biopsy after noting the abnormal size of my left ovary, or microscopically examine the fluid from the cyst? Why didn't at least one of my numerous doctors order a CA-125 earlier in my disease? If any of these procedures had occurred, early intervention would most probably have had me cured and back to normal. Did I contribute to my delayed diagnosis by using natural progesterone and masking my symptoms? I even went so far as to ask the head of gynaecology and obstetrics at the hospital I attended if I had a case for negligence against my original surgeon, and he said I did. I discussed with my children the possibility of suing, but finally decided I wanted to leave the past behind me and concentrate on a happy, healthy future.

What angers me most is the injury to my back, a twisted sacrum, probably sustained during anaesthetic, by not putting both my legs in the stirrups at the same time prior to my curette. It is an ongoing problem that has cost me a lot of money for treatment, and much discomfort and limitation on my daily living ever since. What I am most grateful for are the two dedicated and very thorough surgeons who spent three-and-a-half hours exploring my abdominal cavity and removing as much cancer as was surgically possible. Their constant postoperative visits and obvious concern for my family and myself was most heartening and appreciated.

My recovery was neither smooth nor routine. The massive wounds healed well, but as soon as I drank anything, I vomited. This necessitated the passing of a tube via my nose, into my stomach, a hideous procedure. The intravenous needle (IV) was reinserted so many times it was an ongoing nightmare for me and the young residents. Three weeks later I was still on IV therapy and not tolerating solid food, and I weighed 43kgs. Any type of solid food caused severe colic, but numerous x-rays revealed there was not a bowel obstruction. Two days before my discharge on June 2nd, the IV was removed and I tolerated a light diet. I looked like a starving refugee with my skinny arms and legs and potbelly, but how happy I was to get out into the fresh air again. I was instructed to return to see the surgeon in two weeks time to arrange chemotherapy.

As Ted was having the preliminary examination before the removal of his cataracts, it had been arranged that Greg pick me up from hospital. At Katrina's insistence, and I must say my relief, I was to convalesce with her in Byawatha. Greg first took me home to collect some clothes and personal belongings, then to visit Mum who had prepared soup and sandwiches for the drive to Katrina's. I really enjoyed the trip and was feeling well and happy. Thomas greeted me with enthusiasm and joined us for a short walk before Greg headed back home.

Dinner was a lovely home-cooked meal of feather-light gnocchi and vegetables, before I settled into Thomas's room for the night. Katrina and Rob's home is an old rammed-earth, four-roomed cottage, so sharing with

Thomas was the only option, and he didn't seem to mind at all. It was so dark and quiet after three weeks in hospital, that when I awoke at 4am with severe abdominal pain, I was quite disorientated.

Later that morning I rang the hospital, and the nurse on duty advised taking laxative tablets. Katrina drove the 40km round trip into Wangaratta to get them for me, but the pain got progressively worse, and my abdomen became more distended. Katrina massaged it for me, which gave some short-term relief, and then she rang the naturopath whose advice was to apply a caster oil compress.

The diarrhoea started at 5pm, accompanied by excruciating pain, and got progressively worse as the evening went by. Katrina took me into Wangaratta Base Hospital five hours later after finding a babysitter for Thomas (Rob was on night shift). I was put back on IV therapy and admitted. Poor Katrina was so distressed, and must have wondered if she'd made the right decision about caring for me.

The staff at Wangaratta Hospital were exceptional, and I appreciated being put into an empty two-bed room. The diarrhoea was finally controlled with medication the next day and a sample collected for culture and sensitivity to antibiotics. The dietitian visited me and prescribed a low-residue diet, and a supplement that was absorbed high in my digestive tract as my inflamed lower bowel was not functioning properly, as well as Yakult to replace the good bacteria to aid digestion and absorption. I wonder now why all this was not done at the other hospital, thus avoiding this setback.

Katrina visited twice a day, running herself ragged, and I worried about her, but Thomas thought visiting hospital was great, and spent his time intrigued with all the hardware concerned with adjusting the bed.

Katrina also arranged for a masseuse, Trisha Scott, to visit me. A very special person entered my life that day, a friend and therapist who has had a huge influence on my physical, emotional and spiritual healing. I will never be able to find the words to express my gratitude to her. She was the key to my new life. On this particular occasion she massaged my feet, which I found very relaxing, and that night I enjoyed a good night's sleep for the first time in over three weeks.

The diarrhoea returned the following day, Friday, and was once again controlled. Katrina had given Ted and the family the latest news, but I had no communication from Ted. Out of the blue that evening, my dear friend of long standing, Bob, who had read to me from the primary readers in the other hospital, arrived to visit. He is one of the most kind-hearted and generous people I know, and I really appreciated his driving up from Melbourne. Ours was a very special relationship, dating back to the mid '60s when Bob and my first husband had worked together, and our families enjoyed socializing. I guess he was a substitute for the estranged brother I hadn't seen since the children were small. Bob and I hadn't seen much of each other since my family's move to the country in the late '70s, but we'd always kept in touch, and been there for each other when it mattered. I had sometimes wondered if it could have been more than that if circumstances had been different.

Bob stayed in a hotel in Wangaratta, as it was the Queen's birthday long weekend. Greg and Jane had arranged with Katrina to bring Wim's body - which the vet had kept frozen - up for burial in her garden. I begged and beseeched, and was given a couple of hours day leave from the hospital on Saturday afternoon, and Bob took me out for the burial and family gathering, and had me back in time for tea.

By Monday I had my first normal bowel action, small, but significant. On Tuesday, the doctor visited armed with the pathology result, and ordered antibiotics for a particularly virulent bug, and discharged me. Katrina and a very excited Thomas picked me up at midday, and I arrived back at the cottage to relax on the verandah with a cuppa - bliss.

Katrina was most conscientious with my diet and supplement, and my insides settled down to a more normal routine. For a special treat she cooked us lamb cutlets for dinner on Thursday, a mutual favorite, but I suffered internally as a consequence: it would turn out to be my last meal of red meat.

Friday 13th June. A far from unlucky day for me, I started the day with a full massage at Trisha's rooms, a wonderfully relaxing birthday gift from Katrina and Rob, then I visited the naturopath, Liz. She pointed out the black spot on my iridology printout that represented the cancer, as well as the signs of a clogged lymphatic system and liver. She advised a very strict diet excluding caffeine, dairy, wheat, egg yolks, yeast products and meat. I was to eat fish three times a week, plus flaxseed oil, barley grass powder with my freshly made fruit and vegetable juices, and double strength antioxidant tablets.

It was all rather overwhelming, but with Katrina's support and inventive cooking, and my determination to be well again, we followed this regime conscientiously. Day by day I gained strength and weight, and unrestricted time with Thomas gave me great joy. A very special bond was forged with my grandson in those weeks and months of living so closely, a bond we still have today, and I hope will continue as he grows up, oh so fast. He is so sweet and loving, always generous with his hugs and kisses, the sweetest joy for a grandmother. The peace, beauty and fresh country air of Byawatha soothed my soul and brought me peace.

To help Katrina, I became chief dishwasher and did any jobs I was physically able to do.

Facing Reality.

Although I was resolved in my own mind that my marriage to Ted was over, I still had to convince him. I wrote a long, kind but firm letter, explaining my feelings and the reasons for my decision to separate. He received it on our wedding anniversary, which was not my intention, and was naturally upset. He rang, begging me to reconsider, and swearing he could and would change, but I told him it was too late.

Ted's cataract operations were a great success, which made driving less hazardous, a relief all round, but he still lacked the incentive to re-channel his energy and talent to fill his time. He kept ringing me up for advice or to abuse me, and I found the emotional confrontations resulting from these telephone exchanges between us exhausting and depressing, and was often reduced to tears.

Having decided to go it alone, the question was where and how I would live.

Katrina and Rob had agreed to allow me to have a granny flat erected on the farm, not too close, but close enough for convenience. I rang the local council and inquired about rules and regulations, and some commercial outlets about the cost of second hand units. This made me feel a little more secure, as the future looked pretty scary at times.

Increasing peace of mind, and the weekly massages I was indulging in, had me sleeping better than I had in years, which must have helped my healing, and my back was pain free at that time.

Percy's Powder

Since discharge from hospital I had been hearing from several sources about 'Percy's Powder'. Some were personal anecdotes from people in the district, and another from a friend of Mum's. There had also been a feature on the local TV news about Percy and his powder, and several people with advanced cancer and no medical treatment options left, were interviewed. They had been using Percy's regime of powder and diet for some time, and were certainly looking well, and had a quality of life and health the doctors couldn't explain. There was, of course, the usual counter argument that 'there was no scientific evidence to prove the validity of this treatment, etc, etc.'

At the time I met him, Percy Weston was an elderly gentleman (over 90), living in Eurobin, near Myrtleford in Northeast Victoria. From what I remember him telling me, he started studying medicine as a young man, but had to discontinue his studies to help on the family farm. In the 1930s he discovered from experience that an over-rigorous application of super phosphate fertilizer to his paddocks over five years, caused leukemia, arthritis and reduced lambing rates in his sheep. He sold 100 of these miserable beasts to a fellow farmer in Myrtleford and watched them recover and thrive on non-super treated pasture, and that started him thinking. Repeated experiments over thirty years showed him that the element responsible for the cause of cancer in his sheep, was phosphorus.

Percy had not only been liberal with super on his paddocks, but also on his farm produce, and paid the penalty in the early 1940s by developing a very painful and inoperable growth. He is confident that he is alive today because of the course of treatment he subsequently devised, and that the way to prevent or cure cancer is to restrict, control and neutralize phosphorus.

He believes that the constant use of soluble phosphoric fertilizers can tie up the calcium, iron, magnesium, potassium and sodium in soils before a plant can utilize them, causing foods to become chronically short of these elements while being saturated with phosphorus. In human nutrition, this phosphorus can be quickly absorbed and integrated into the bloodstream, and in the form of adenosine triphosphate (ATP), has the power to penetrate any cell of the body. If the other nutrient elements are not present in sufficient quantities in the extra-cellular fluids to maintain a balance, the ATP will commandeer those elements from the intra-cellular fluids to heal sick or injured tissue and produce an inversion of procedures that leads to cancer.

Percy supplies comprehensive lists of foods and their phosphorus content, and a list of the contents of his powder in their percentages, and what each element is for.

He recommends that the powder be taken at bedtime at least three hours after the evening meal. The aim is to allow the formula to have control of the body for a prolonged period of time through the hours of sleep and rest. The average dose is 1/2 a teaspoon dissolved in a tall glass of cold water, to which is added the juice of half a lemon, which makes a pleasant fizzy drink like fruit saline. Deep breathing before bedtime to fill the blood stream with oxygen, and a copious drink of cold water on rising are also recommended in conjunction with the powder.

Percy states that two or three months are usually required before the cancerous growth shrivels and is absorbed by the rest of the body. The cure is simple to apply, painless and inexpensive. "The cure of cancer and the like is thus made possible by my invention; in short, I reverse the nature of the chemical intake which is the cause of the condition," says Percy.

Percy also believes that it would be possible to make his formula up in a tablet form, which could be used as indicated with the correct diet. There is also a group of herbs, which have an almost identical analysis, but for Percy, an even more promising prospect is the group of seaweeds - dulce, agar, kelp, and irishmoss - whose chemical content is eminently suitable for the same purpose, which could also prove effective if used in tablet form with correct diet.

To my knowledge, these are dreams of Percy's as yet unfulfilled, but not from want of trying. A truly remarkable, warm and caring man.

With all this information at hand, I decided to start taking Percy's Powder at his recommended ¼ teaspoon dose (because of my low weight). Rather than struggle with the extensive lists of do's and don'ts with food items (my diet was complicated enough), I decided to eat as much organically grown food as possible. We had always grown our own vegetables, and Katrina had a number of fruit trees, and was planting more.

We found a commercial outlet for the other organic food basics, and although not perfect, we were happy that we were eliminating as much phosphorus-saturated food as possible from our diet. My general health continued to improve.

Back to Healesville.

Wednesday the 25th of June. I reluctantly traveled back to Healesville and Ted, as I couldn't put off a visit to my surgeon to discuss chemotherapy any longer. I had already cancelled one appointment, as I wanted extra time to gain weight and strength. On crossing the mountains, we left the sunshine behind and descended into the damp and cold. The weather matched perfectly my reception by Ted.

There was no food in the house, so I had to go shopping. The garden was miserably neglected, the vacuum cleaner had obviously been on extended holiday, and the sheets hadn't been changed since I went to hospital.

Ted acted as if I had changed my mind and come back for good, but when it was made clear to the contrary, he started ranting and threatening suicide. When he said he'd leave and stay with his younger daughter Debbie, I just hoped he meant it.

I had a bath and tried to relax, realizing I was back in the same hellhole.

Arising early after a sleepless night, I went to see the surgeon who had operated on me. He was very pleasantly surprised at how well I was, expecting me to have jaundice and ascites (fluid in the abdominal cavity). He had already made an appointment with the gyn/oncologist at the Mercy Hospital for Women in Melbourne for the following day; he was very keen for me to start chemotherapy as soon as possible. *(See Appendix 2, 'Treatment Choices')*

On arriving home, I baked and did a load of washing and rang the family while Ted rested. Who was the sick one here?

Ted insisted on driving me to Melbourne the following afternoon. The traffic was horrendous, and by the time we arrived he was exhausted. I had a long and detailed chat with a very caring gyn/oncologist. Her idea was for me to start chemotherapy the following Thursday, and have treatments every three weeks for six sessions. This necessitated a kidney function test to ascertain the appropriate dosage, and this was arranged for the following Wednesday at a specialist cancer clinic elsewhere in Melbourne. Following blood tests, I rejoined Ted two hours after leaving him.

He had refused to go to the café for refreshments, so by the time he had driven half way home he was feeling faint, and his right leg was so painful I had to take over the driving. It seemed that letting him transport me in the future would be out of the question. The latest news was passed on once more to the families that evening.

Over the weekend I cleaned the house and tidied the worst of the garden while Ted rested and watched the football. He still had hopes for reconciliation, and wanted me to work out what he was to do with his life. Both Joan and Margot rang, and Joan offered to transport me to the Mercy the following Thursday for chemotherapy, which I gratefully accepted. Ted protested and said it was 'his duty,' but I stood firm, not needing the added stress.

Katrina rang for a chat Sunday morning and asked if I had changed my mind about leaving Ted, and was most relieved when assured I hadn't. Several years earlier, when his manic episodes had become so violent and uncontrolled that I feared for my physical safety, I had left him. I returned when he developed pneumonia as a result of not taking his medication and had refused to go to hospital.

His behavior moderated for quite a few months after that, and I dared to hope we could re-establish a happy and stable relationship, but his condition deteriorated again to the stage it was in 1996.

By Monday, Ted had obviously accepted the situation and started making lists of what belonged to whom, reclaiming any items he'd contributed to the house, and any gifts he had given me, including my rings, which I refused to surrender.

Exhausted from all the stress, I wondered how I could possibly heal in this environment.

Ted's son-in-law Ian, had offered to drop me at the clinic on Wednesday for the kidney test, if I could get myself to their place by the time he left for work at 7.15am. This entailed an early, foggy start, but was a practical solution.

Arriving safely, I commenced the procedure at 9.15, and it was completed by early afternoon, then Bob drove me back to my car at Ringwood. I rang Joan that evening to finalize arrangements for the next day, before retiring early, tired out.

My Chemotherapy Begins.

From talking to other cancer patients and oncology nurses, and from my reading, I am aware that everyone has a unique reaction to chemotherapy. Some have a minimum of discomfort and side effects, while others are severely debilitated, and everything in-between. I have always been sensitive to drugs, so my reaction was relative to that. *(See Appendix 3, 'How Chemotherapy Works')*

Thursday 3rd July. First Chemotherapy treatment.

I arose early and kept myself busy, doing two loads of washing, cleaning the bathrooms and sweeping the floors - my way of coping with the fear and uncertainty - until Joan picked me up just after nine.

We arrived at the Mercy at 10.30, and Joan went off to the city to fill in the time. She had offered to stay with me, but I had declined, as I was happier on my own with a book and my Walkman for distraction.

It took the nurse three attempts to get the IV into my damaged veins, then I had to wait until one o'clock for the first bag of chemo to arrive, then another wait before the second one was put up. The staff were in gowns and protective eyewear, and double gloved. What was I doing to myself? I had always been so fussy about the quality of food and beverage I consumed, and until late '96, rarely took any medication, and now I was allowing my body to be filled with deadly poisons. I felt so scared and out of control that I just wanted to run out of there, and keep running, leaving the whole hideous nightmare behind me. Why was this happening to me? Why, why, why?

When Joan picked me up I was feeling dizzy and washed out. She had trouble hiding her concern at my condition and appearance, which must have added to the stress of coping with peak hour traffic. What a dear friend.

I felt ghastly and lay down for a while after arriving home. Ted watched TV and ate the meal I had prepared for him as if all was normal. The vomiting started around seven that evening. The anti-nausea tablets the hospital had sent home with me had no affect, but a suppository for the same purpose eventually took effect and I went to bed. I woke a couple of times and dry retched, and then slept until after midnight. I needed something in my stomach, so I had some fruit juice. I read for a while and then slept until morning. I made porridge for our breakfast and enjoyed it, but then went back to bed, as the morning was so cold.

Katrina rang to say she was on her way down, and I rang Mum to assure her I was okay. My sister Brenda also rang to see how I was.

Ted was very nasty about the fact that Katrina was coming, so when she and Thomas arrived and I was not feeling too bad, the three of us took a picnic lunch to Maroondah Dam where we could talk in peace and Thomas could run around. We went and saw Mum on our way home, and filled the evening with a video, though

Ted still managed to slip in the odd snide remark. Thank goodness he was going to stay with his daughter for a few days.

It was freezing cold the following day, so Katrina, Thomas and I spent the morning at a nice warm shopping centre, though I found the outing tiring.

We came home for lunch and lit the fire. Ted finally left mid afternoon, clearing the air so we could relax. Mum came over and sat by the fire and we had a lovely chat, three generations of women in harmony, love and support together; why couldn't life be full of such simple pleasures?

Mum hadn't had the opportunity to spend a lot of time with Thomas, so it was a special time for them as well. I cooked dinner for us, but nausea ruined my appetite and I couldn't eat it and just had a little yogurt and stewed apple instead.

A restless night was followed by a morning so cold the water pipes froze, so we sat over breakfast until they thawed. Katrina dug up some raspberry plants and picked lemons to take back home. She filled the wood box for me, as I was feeling too weak and shaky to do much. She and Thomas headed home at lunchtime and I sobbed with self-pity.

I was starting to have second thoughts about going on with chemotherapy.

I don't know why I hated it so much. Was it just how sick it made me feel, or the thought of my whole body being poisoned? According to medical opinion it was the best option for prolonging my life, but how important was that? I was probably going to die soon anyway, so why put myself through this, just postponing the inevitable? I'd fulfilled most of my dreams; my childhood fantasies of dancing on my toes, of being a nurse, having babies; my adolescent goals of love, husband, home and family; my adult dreams of flying, a farm and my beloved donkeys. I'd seen my children mature, succeed in their careers, choose a partner, and I had a beautiful grandchild. The future spent alone, unemployed, and on a limited income after finalising my marriage, seemed daunting.

Okay, I still had a few unfulfilled plans – to see Central and Northern Australia and the Great Barrier Reef; to hang glide – but how important were they?

Then I thought of my wonderful family, the anguish, love and worry on Mum's face, knowing as a mother myself, how terrible it would be for her to see her child die. The horror, helplessness and bewilderment on my children's faces as they contemplated losing a parent too soon.

Katrina had already put so much effort into my care, and was practically willing me to stay alive, and I was just getting to know darling Thomas. If I didn't hang on for quite a bit longer, he wouldn't even remember me.

But I HATE chemo!

Not being one to wallow in self pity for any length of time, I rang Liz, my naturopath, and had a chat about my reaction and thoughts about chemo, and she offered to send me some homeopathic drops to help me detoxify more quickly. I also rang the Gawler Foundation and left a message. The Foundation is located at Yarra Junction, and was originally run by Dr Ian and Grace Gawler. It is a charitable group providing active support for cancer patients and their families. It also promotes health and well-being throughout the community. You may attend on a daily basis or as a resident.

I re-read some of Ian Gawler's book, which answered

some of my questions. I had smaller, more frequent meals to avoid nausea, and enjoyed a lovely peaceful evening alone by the fire.

Following a good night's sleep - at last - the next morning was not so cold. I rang the social worker at the Mercy who had offered her services if ever I needed them, and discussed the possibility of having my remaining chemotherapy sessions at Wangaratta Hospital. I felt in need of care and support during further treatment, and Katrina was offering that if I stayed with her. I couldn't see it happening at home with Ted. The social worker said she would see what she could do, and ring me back the following Wednesday.

The Gawler Foundation returned my call and I arranged to visit there the following Monday for counselling and meditation. I indulged in a restful day to nurse a sore throat. I was not able to eat much, but I managed to keep up fluid and fruit.

I rang Ted to see how his weekend at the football had gone, and also rang Bob for a nice chat, something I couldn't do when Ted was home, and continued my internal debate whether or not to go on with chemo.

Reality strikes

My part-pension was proving inadequate and my funds were running low. I decided to try and cash the small amount of superannuation I had acquired over 2 ½ years as a pharmacy assistant but needed a doctor to fill in a form. It was rather a shock when my GP described my disease on the required form as 'advanced' ovarian cancer, with a 6 – 20 month life expectancy. All these terms are familiar to me now, but surprisingly, that was the first time my condition really struck home. It certainly gave me food for thought, and some occasions of regret and deep depression. How dare anyone presume to put a time expectation on another person's life? We all have our own journey to make, in our own way. The seed was sown for my determination to blow the medical profession's statistics out of the water!

Before returning home, I did some shopping for Ted and Mum's forthcoming birthdays, and had my hair cut, which cheered me up. This was possibly the last visit to a hairdresser before the chemo caused my hair to fall out, something I absolutely dreaded.

I had some phone calls and an unexpected visitor in the evening, which was pleasant and diverting, but I was still undecided whether to go on with chemotherapy.

The next couple of days were spent quietly, nursing my cold and relaxing. The social worker had rung to tell me she'd been able to arrange for my on-going chemotherapy at Wangaratta, and the oncologist rang later to confirm this, as long as I came back to the Mercy for my fifth treatment.

Ted arrived home unexpectedly on Thursday afternoon. I was not pleased, and he picked up the feeling and sulked all night. It did not improve his mood when he learnt I was going back to Byawatha the following Tuesday, but what choice did I have?

On Monday, I was due at the Gawler Foundation. The Yarra Valley Living Centre as it is called, is set in bushland in a peaceful valley. The grounds have lots of quiet places to sit and enjoy the tranquillity.

I had a very supportive and encouraging session with the counsellor, then joined the meditation group. I felt quite robust compared with many of the group members, some without hair, which reminded me what was possibly in store in the not too distant future. I did manage to relax and participate to a certain degree, but it was all so new and strange to me.

I decided to buy a set of Ian Gawler's meditation tapes to enable me to practice on my own. I also purchased a detailed book on juices, as I felt they were an important part of my detoxification, a natural and concentrated way of obtaining lots of antioxidants, and an excellent book called '*Cancer as a Turning Point*' by Lawrence Leshan. How beneficial it must be to attend a residential course there.

I was home by lunchtime and spent some time with Mum, sharing my morning's experience with her. Such a wise woman, well and broadly read, her mind open to all possibilities and theories. A good listener, she has firm views of her own but never tries to force them on others. How I would miss our precious times together. It was so hard leaving her alone in Healesville, but we both knew I was making the right decision to leave my old life behind, and seek healing of my body, mind and spirit in the Northeast, which I have long loved.

I made Ted his usual chocolate birthday cake, knowing it would be for the last time.

Tuesday 15th July was Ted's birthday, and the official going of our separate ways, as he had arranged to spend the day with his family. Katrina, Rob and Thomas were calling in on their way home from a rare short break at Cowes, Phillip Island, then I would travel to Byawatha with them in convoy.

Not surprisingly, Ted showed no enthusiasm for his gift, card and cake. I busied myself with last minute washing, which was put in the dryer, vacuumed the house, and packed. Ted had left by late morning, very upset, declaring it the worst birthday of his life.

Poor Ted. It wasn't that I hated him; I had just put a barrier around my feelings towards him for my own protection. I had tried numerous times to explain, but he just wouldn't hear me. He believed in nothing but himself and what he could see, touch, own and control. I had been one of the very few people in his life whom he had trusted and respected, and in his eyes I had betrayed him. What he saw as his world and his life was disintegrating, and it must have been frightening.

I knew his family was planning a celebration, but I didn't think his heart would be in it. I did feel very sad for him, a victim of his disturbed mind, but I also felt a huge weight lift from my shoulders, and a great freedom of spirit as he drove away.

A New Life

My little family arrived just as I finished packing the car. They had recently stopped for lunch, so we lost no time heading north. I had said a difficult and tearful farewell to Mum earlier. She looked so forlorn and alone as she waved us goodbye.

Katrina travelled in my car with me to share the driving, but I drove all the way with just a petrol stop, I was feeling so good. On arrival at the cottage, we got the fires going and unpacked the cars, then we were all ready for an early night.

Once I had recovered from the after effects of my first dose of chemotherapy, and was feeling more secure in Katrina's care, I decided to continue with the treatment.

During the week prior to the next session, I needed to have the required blood tests and meet the local physician charged with the supervision of the chemotherapy and my hospital stay. I requested staying overnight in the hospital so my restlessness and vomiting wouldn't disturb Thomas or worry Katrina.

I'm sure the doctor was perfectly competent, but I didn't

exactly warm to him. He dismissed my theory that the stress of living with a manic depressant for five years may have contributed to my illness. It has been well documented, and is quite widely accepted these days, that prolonged stress can have a detrimental affect on a person's health and well-being. Psychiatrist, Dr Ainslie Meares, was a pioneer in this field, and has had his theories verified. His credo was that, 'We have an immune system that fights cancer; we have a hormone – cortisone – that inhibits the immune system's action. And we know that more cortisone flows when stress, anxiety and tension are at their most acute stage. And that gives cancer a free run.'

Dr Ann Wooley-Hart of London, who had cancer herself ten years before, and was working along similar lines to Ainslie Meares, states, 'Stress from whatever cause raises the level of circulating corticosteroids with resulting depression of immune functions.' Two American researchers, Doctors Carl Simonton and Stephanie Matthews-Simonton, have also investigated the role that stress plays in malignancy. 'Emotional depression in reaction to stress seems to result in physical depression of the body's immune system, and that permits the growth of malignancy.' These are just a few examples of early research results.

My physician also considered my complementary therapies a waste of time and money. Not an auspicious start. Luckily, the local GP I would later consult was a warm and caring lady, and very supportive.

I also revisited Trisha Scott to have the tension massaged out of my neck and shoulders.

I kept in touch with Ted by phone, but he was most unresponsive. He had wasted no time in going to a solicitor and rewriting his will, and putting the house on the market. He refused to spend his money on food, so he alternated between his daughters for meals, and they sent him home with meals on plates ready to be reheated. Ted soon abandoned living on his own altogether, and spent most of his time with either of his daughters.

Rob was able to fix a couple of problems I was having with my old car, and my days were spent working in the garden with Katrina, helping about the house, and of course, lots of fun with Thomas. We discovered all sorts of insects and interesting rocks together, and he 'helped' with the weeding. I even assisted Rob, and his dad Graham, with the cattle, a steep learning curve, and started feeling like a real country girl again. It intrigued me the way Graham could always identify each individual cow and calf, even when they were milling around in a confused mob in the yards. He had farmed in the district his whole life, and had a wonderful rapport with all the animals in his charge.

Daily meditation with the help of the tapes was most relaxing, and seemed to clear my mind and soothe my emotions.

Dr Ian Gawler practiced and taught the form of meditation he had originally learnt from Dr Ainslie Meares. For a full explanation of Dr Meares original theory and methods, read his book '*Relief Without Drugs*'. In summary, Dr Meares explains, 'If we can learn to relax physically, we can use the ease of the body to promote a calm mind. … It is in the stillness of the mind that the brain comes to integrate the excessive sensory input. Mental equilibrium is restored and anxiety reduced.'

To experience complete physical relaxation, he led his patients in progressive relaxation of muscle groups, which had the effect of keeping the mind alert. 'As we come to experience our relaxation, it is not so much that our body is relaxed, but that we are relaxed. Our whole self. More than our body and our mind. Our whole being. Stillness comes, not all at once, at first momentarily and fleetingly, then for longer periods.'

When Ian Gawler came to Ainslie Meares in the mid 1970s, he had cancerous bony lumps protruding from his ribs, and his leg had been amputated. His doctors told him that the lumps would double in size for every month he lived (which was not expected to be many). Ian said he believed his cancer was the physical manifestation of disharmony within. 'If people listened to themselves they would learn the lesson that their disease was trying to teach them. I think the disease is the end stage of your soul trying to tell you something is wrong.'

He followed Dr Meares intense and prolonged meditation course, and in 1985, with no sign of cancer in his body, he was leading his own cancer support group. He said, 'For me, the keys to unlocking a patients' ability to help themselves are meditation, positive thinking, dietary principles and support: stress management included.'

(For full details of Ian's story, read '*You Can Conquer Cancer*'.)

I spent time on the verandah meditating and reading some inspiring books I had been lent, including one by Bernie Siegal called '*Peace, Love and Healing: the path to self-healing*'. As a consequence, as my treatment day approached I was feeling much calmer about chemo than I had expected.

Wednesday 23rd July was the day for my second dose of chemotherapy, my first at Wangaratta Base Hospital Oncology Unit, and it was a totally different experience. There were just four patients and the most wonderful oncology nurse you could ever hope to meet. I think she could find a vein in a pumpkin! After explaining the trouble I had with nausea and vomiting last time, she gave me the strongest anti-emetic drug without hesitation. Her attitude was "nothing is too good for my cancer patients, no matter the cost."

The horrible groggy feeling I had experienced after my first chemo session didn't recur, and I even had a little lunch and tea. I found out at a later date that I had been over-dosed on the first occasion, as they hadn't waited for the renal function result to calculate my dose. Instead they had given me the average dose, which turned out to be too much.

On completion, I was shown to a ward and spent the afternoon and evening in an armchair in the day room, reading. I couldn't believe how good I was feeling, but sleep evaded me, so I was given a sleeping pill and was still a bit dopey when Katrina took me home next morning, after only one bout of vomiting. I couldn't get warm, but after some fruit and a snooze on the couch by the fire, I felt better, and went for a short walk and meditated.

I was able to take it easy for the next couple of days and read. I meditated and snoozed between small, nourishing meals and juices, which kept the nausea pretty much at bay.

By Sunday I was feeling good enough to go out with Katrina and Rob to collect firewood. We lit a barbecue in the paddock for lunch, which Thomas loved, but I was glad of a rest by the afternoon.

While I was alone in the house on Monday, Ted rang full of gloom and doom. He was not feeling well and asked if we were getting together again, and when I said no, he got nasty.

I then had to ring the Department of Social Security (DSS), to start the process of getting a disability pension, as Ted had informed them we were separated, and I was no longer entitled to a wife-pension.

On a brighter note, Greg rang to say he'd booked a joy flight out of Wangaratta Airfield for the following Saturday. It was Greg and Jane's belated birthday gift to me, and they were coming to stay for the weekend. I enjoyed helping Rob and his dad, Graham, with the calves that afternoon.

I awoke the next day with backache and sciatica again; I thought that was behind me, and was most disappointed. That was followed by an abusive phone call from Ted, which caused me to break down crying. I rang him back later and forbade him to ring me again except in an emergency. The remainder of the day was spent resting to relieve my back.

Trisha massaged my back the next day, which helped a lot. At the time, we were having a run of frosty mornings followed by warm, sunny days, which were conducive to relaxing on the verandah, so I made the most of it, hoping to be fit for the weekend.

Greg and Jane arrived Friday evening, and we were up early the following morning, thanks to an excited Thomas. We arrived at the airfield at eleven, in perfect weather. Katrina, Thomas and I went on the first flight over Wangaratta, to Byawatha and the surrounding hills: Thomas was thrilled. Greg and Jane came on the second circuit with me; it was Jane's first small plane flight. What a great birthday present. We all then adjourned to a local pub for lunch, and as it had a playground keeping Thomas happily occupied, Katrina could relax and enjoy her meal. Later in the day, Greg did some basic maintenance on my car, and some jobs for his sister, while we girls made pizzas for tea.

We sat over breakfast on Sunday, then we all went fishing, with no luck but lots of fun, then Greg and Jane headed home. If it weren't for my aching back, it would have been a perfect weekend.

I saw Trisha for a massage the next day, and her diagnosis was that I had a twisted sacrum and an inflamed left kidney. She worked on my back for an hour. Liz was also at the rooms, and gave me some anti-inflammatory drops.

The next few days were spent quietly, limited by the back pain, so on Thursday I rang Trisha and asked her opinion about seeing a chiropractor. She knew of one she could recommend, who she consequently rang to discuss my case. Katrina took me to see him in the afternoon, and he made some gentle adjustments. As I was impressed by his caring attitude, I made an appointment to see him again the following Tuesday.

We had a thunderstorm that evening, the first Thomas remembers, and he talked about the 'big boom' long after it had abated. Over an inch (25mm) of much-needed rain fell overnight: the paddocks were visibly greening by the following afternoon.

By Saturday my back was feeling a lot better, so I decided to make bread. I have always loved doing it, and made all our bread when the children were young and we lived on our hobby farm. It was also good upper body exercise, and part of my get-fit program. The resulting loaf smelt and tasted delicious.

On Sunday, Rob was home, so we three adults put in a joint effort to prepare a garden bed for asparagus and berries. We even got the planting done and celebrated with fish and chips and a drink at our local pub, The Tavern, in El Dorado. I've been told it's the smallest pub in the Southern Hemisphere. I met some of the locals, who were very friendly.

Monday morning was spent in Wangaratta, where I had

a massage and went to pathology for my pre-chemo blood tests. I also inquired about a solicitor specializing in family law, as Ted insisted we settle our finances legally ASAP. I also enrolled at the Community Centre for a Tai Chi class, and booked a seat on a bus trip to Mt Macedon for a day to look at gardens, in the company of one of Katrina's neighbours, Anna. I was re-claiming my life.

All this diversion was not enough to stop negative thoughts about my approaching chemotherapy session. It seemed I was just starting to feel well and take charge of my life, and I would be knocked down again. A downward spiral to depression began. I was feeling the need for privacy, and it was becoming obvious that Rob was too, though he always tried to be polite and accommodating. The atmosphere was tense when he was home, and I cried myself to sleep that night.

Katrina and Rob were both working the next day, and I got the weeps again in the morning thinking about chemo making me sick the next day, just as my back was starting to improve. I was wallowing in self-pity, needing my own space and feeling like a parasite. A phone call to Bob resulted in an offer to come and pick me up and take me to visit some friends of his with a holiday home at Venus Bay, for the weekend. I jumped at the opportunity and arranged to postpone chemo for a week.

I also rang Liz, and she suggested writing down all my negative feelings, especially about Ted, then taking the paper outside to burn in a plant pot, watching my problems dissipate with the smoke. I did so, and it was certainly therapeutic. Feeling in a better mood, I set to and did two loads of washing, and made bread and coffee scrolls (Rob's favourites), to celebrate.

When she got home, I explained to Katrina how I felt, and though upset, she understood. I had an adjustment with the chiropractor in the afternoon, and he was pleased with my progress.

Escape

The following morning Katrina drove me to Bonnie Doon, the halfway point where Bob met us, and after a picnic lunch we went our separate ways. Bob drove me to the Mercy Hospital where I had an appointment with the gyn/oncologist, but it had been written in for the wrong day, so we went on to his place. Later that day I received a phone call with the blood test results; all back to normal, including renal function, and my CA-125 was down to 18 (below 15 is considered negative). This result gave me the incentive I needed to continue with the course of chemo, as it was obviously working.

A simple meal with a glass of wine to celebrate, followed by a soaking bath before bed, ended a long but satisfying day.

The following day we visited Bob's daughter Rebecca and her children, and later watched the movie, *'The Castle'*. Laughter certainly is good medicine. We ended the day with dinner at Greg and Jane's and more laughter.

On Friday, Bob and I visited more friends from when our children were young, Robert and Isabel. (Their youngest son is my godson). They are such special people, for after having three children of their own, they fostered dozens more, adopting one of them. Isabel had her own health problems, including chronic kidney disease, but undaunted, they battled on together, still fostering. We had lost touch over the years, but Bob had told them of my illness when I was in hospital, and they had visited several times. With friends like that, time apart doesn't seem to matter.

Over several cups of tea I explained my feelings, and they offered to bring their caravan to Byawatha in a few weeks time, and set it up in the backyard of the cottage. This would give us all some extra space and privacy. I jumped at the idea, although it would only be until January as they were planning a holiday in the caravan. Life was looking brighter all round.

The family that was hosting our stay at Venus Bay was struck down with gastroenteritis, so that trip was off, but Bob and I decided to head for the coast anyway. We stopped at Cape Patterson for a walk along the beach. Bob isn't a great one for exercise, so I wandered alone among the rocks. I sat down and gazed out to sea, savouring the fresh salty air in my face, the constant mew of seagulls, the lullaby of the waves, and the distinctive smell of the seaside. I didn't want to leave this beautiful world. What if this were the last time I saw the sea, walked along the beach? Why did this disease have to happen to me?

Death held no fears for me, just the process of dying, but I had too much living still to do. What were my beliefs? I had rejected the idea of heaven and hell and a vengeful, judging God watching over my every thought, and making notes in an eternal book; yes, as a child this is what I had learnt and believed. It was certainly a practical way to try and make me a 'good girl'. But through a journey of living, listening and studying, I was at a stage of believing there was some sort of higher force, and that our lives had meaning and direction, and that we were free to make choices and live and learn from the consequences. I was confident that the essential element of who we are continues after earthly death, and I was even open to the possibility of reincarnation. My practical nature precluded accepting that the experience and lessons of this life were for nothing. It was not something I spent time and deep thought contemplating, but my basic philosophy for many years had been that if life didn't include loving, learning and growing, it wasn't worth having. That was before I actually looked death in the face.

After a little cry, I rejoined Bob and we enjoyed a Chinese meal. Bob's car had developed a strange noise and a warning light had come on, so we abandoned further plans for recreation and headed back to his place. We then faced the dilemma of alternative transport to get me back to Wangaratta for the next chemotherapy session. Greg came to the rescue and lent us his ute, as he was flying back to Darwin for the next three weeks to work and could do without it.

We were on the way north by 9.30 the next morning. We bought some bakery goodies in Wangaratta for lunch to share with Katrina, and then Bob headed back home. I drove into Wangaratta later for a chiropractic appointment and a therapeutic chat with Liz, then topped up on vitamins, and went to DSS to find my disability pension had been approved.

Tuesday was to be the last day I expected to be feeling well for a week or more, so I helped out by washing, ironing and baking. I had a rest and read in the afternoon, then made naan bread to have with an Indian meal Katrina had prepared. I received phone calls from Mum, Greg and Bob in the evening, letting me know they'd be thinking of me over the next few days. How loved I felt.

Chemotherapy day dawned again, marking the halfway point of my treatment. Time to put into action some of what I had been learning and practising. I tried to direct my thoughts away from the negative and see the drugs as allies attacking and defeating the cancer cells; it took a lot of concentration.

The day passed without mishap, but I had a bad night with nausea and an irritated bladder. I vomited before discharge the next morning, but after Katrina had brought me back to the cottage, I slept on the sun lounge until lunchtime. Another snooze in the afternoon restored me.

Thomas had his first hair cut.

My usual week of lethargy and nausea followed. Washing my hair one morning, I looked down and saw the plughole clogged with a thick wad of my hair. Bursting into tears, I gently patted my hair dry. My worst nightmare was becoming reality, despite following all the advice I'd been given about using a soft hairbrush and baby shampoo. Each morning I expected to find chunks of hair on my pillow, but was only greeted with a profusion of loose hairs. I was very lucky and didn't lose all my hair. It thinned out a lot and lost its color, but as it was normally very thick, no one noticed the thinning but me. I was eternally grateful and couldn't believe my luck. But was it just luck, or had the large doses of antioxidants I consumed in juices, tablets and drops contributed by minimizing the damage to healthy cells and sped their recovery?

Thomas came down with a cold and developed croup a couple of nights later. I was glad to be able to advise Katrina and Rob on what to do, as it is a very frightening experience for both the child and parents.

Tension between Rob and me was increasing. I guessed it was the old problem of 'three's a crowd'. He worked such long hours — twelve-hour shifts at work, plus share-farm cropping and helping his dad with the cattle — that time with his family was precious, and I was an intruder. I tried hiding my unhappiness from Katrina, and stayed in the kitchen while they were in the lounge together as a family. I rang Bob and asked if he could hurry the caravan along.

Being in need of more clothes and personal belongings, Katrina, Thomas and I did a round trip to Healesville one day, knowing Ted would not be there. On arrival, I packed all I wanted and then we visited Mum for a chat and a cuppa.

She was pleasantly surprised to see how well I was looking, which gave her some comfort. I was slowly but surely regaining the weight and muscle lost while in hospital.

We headed back home after lunch, with Thomas clutching the toolbox I had given him containing a few basic tools from when I was between handyman husbands. He was rapt, and didn't let it out of his sight. He even slept that night with the pliers grasped in his little hand! Bob rang that evening to say the caravan would be arriving Friday; hooray!

First step to Independence.

Friday dawned, and I went to pathology, and had a massage prior to the caravan arriving at about four. Rob, Bob and Robert (so confusing!) positioned it, while Isabel and I talked grandchildren. Robert and Isabel headed home after a cuppa, and we persuaded Bob, who had followed in his car, to stay for dinner and the night (he slept in the caravan).

Bob departed for home after a cooked breakfast the next day and I started moving into the caravan. I bought myself a radio/cassette/CD player on my next visit to Wangaratta, for company and entertainment in the caravan, and I also had my first visit to the solicitor. She suggested that a 60/40 split with Ted would be fair and reasonable, and said she would write a letter to that effect to his solicitor, but I didn't expect for a moment he'd agree. I had spent all my money, the total proceeds from the sale of my original house, on the home we shared together. Ted added $20,000 to make up the full amount, but because we were married he considered he had the right to 50% of its value. Knowing him, I guessed he would fight tooth and nail to get what he wanted, whereas I just wanted it settled and over with.

Rob was still very cool towards me, but at least I had the caravan to retreat to. I read, wrote and played my favorite CDs to cheer myself up.

Thomas thought the caravan was a big cubby house, and loved to visit. I continued to help Katrina in the house and garden when Rob wasn't around, and withdrew from their family life as much as possible. Poor Katrina was the meat in the sandwich.

On the evening of Rob's birthday, I ate early before having a bath and retiring to the caravan, leaving them to have a family celebration, but Thomas had trouble understanding why I was not included. I breakfasted alone in the caravan the next morning, the first of many such meals.

Princess Diana was killed, and the world was stunned.

There followed a run of very cold weather. I awoke in the early hours one morning, freezing. I reheated my hot water bottle and put on socks, a hat and an extra blanket, but couldn't get back to sleep. The water in the glass beside my bed froze. Arising at eight, I put on the heater and the kettle and blew the fuse, so went back to bed and cried.

I went over to the house later for boiling water, and Katrina fixed the fuse and told me I was silly to cry, which made me cry more. Later, she picked me some flowers and we hugged and made up.

What an emotional mess I was. In hindsight, I can see that the mood swings, along with the multiple hot flushes and night sweats, were part of my instant menopause following the total hysterectomy. The chemotherapy drugs playing havoc with my normal body function weren't helping either.

Another freezing night followed, with little sleep. I went for a long walk along the creek the next day, and spent the evening in the caravan listening to Diana's funeral.

I felt I would rather be dead than live feeling like a displaced person.

Sunday was a very eventful day, and reminded me that I was still of some use. I was summoned from the caravan by Rob, who was distressed by his fathers' condition; he appeared to be having an asthma attack. Borrowing Katrina's asthma spray, I gave him two puffs and then drove him to the hospital. Rob had to hurry back to the cattle yards to finish pulling a dead calf out of its mother, and Katrina was tied up entertaining her father and stepmother who were on a brief visit from Melbourne. A family member eventually arrived at the hospital to take over Graham's care, and I went back home.

After a late lunch and the departure of the visitors, I was writing letters in the caravan when Katrina asked my advice about Thomas, who was continually vomiting. I considered it a typical childhood attach of gastritis, but suggested she ring the hospital. They said to bring him in, but after 2 ½ hours of trying to comfort a sick child in the casualty department, they confirmed my diagnosis, and we brought him home. I rang Mum later, and she gave me the news that she was having an operation on her face the next day, and was understandably very apprehensive. Once again, I was able to call upon my nursing experience, and gave her advice and reassurance. It eased my mind knowing my sister Brenda would be there to care for her.

That night there was a huge thunderstorm.

Thomas bounced back quickly, as kids do. I wished my old car could do the same. It seemed that every time

I drove it something else broke, and the last time I had to leave it with the mechanic for new belts, I was informed it needed new tie rods – the car would have to wait until after my next chemo session.

After my fourth dose of chemotherapy, I was sicker than ever and needed IV medication in the middle of the night to control the vomiting.

I was pretty wobbly when Katrina picked me up the following morning, and rested most of the day. I was feeling stronger by late afternoon, which was just as well, as Katrina had become ill and needed me to bath Thomas and cook tea. No one was hungry, so after tucking Thomas into bed, I went out to the caravan for an early night.

After she had recovered, Katrina and Thomas went to Melbourne for a few days to catch up with friends. Bob came up for the weekend and we enjoyed a choral recital at Wangaratta Cathedral and a tour of Beechworth and the Millawa gourmet region, very relaxed and comfortable in each others company.

Katrina arrived home about midday the following Thursday looking refreshed and more relaxed. We had a catch-up chat, and she assured me Mum was doing well following her operation.

It didn't take long for tension to mount again. I went over to the house early one Saturday to make myself some toast. The family was having breakfast together, and I was not given a warm welcome; I felt like a leper. Feeling hurt, I ended up weepy and depressed all day. I wrote Katrina a note telling her of my feelings, and she asked me over to the house to talk about it, but I couldn't. Reading and a long walk passed the day, but the evening meal I shared with them was very strained. I just had to get out of there and stop messing up their life together, and get one of my own.

My car was back at the mechanic's on the Monday as planned. That evening, Rob asked me if I would like to go to an agricultural field day at Henty, NSW, with them the next day. Although I had arranged to go to Melbourne, I took it as a peace offering and accepted. Graham came along too, and we were on the road just after seven. It was a glorious sunny day.

There were acres of farm machinery and allied equipment, which the men found absorbing and Thomas had fun climbing all over, but by lunchtime, Katrina and I decided to go off on our own and look at things of more interest to us. That worked well, and Katrina bought herself an Akubra hat, and I got a birthday gift for Brenda and some boot covers for Ted, to stop debris filling his boots when he mowed and used the whipper-snipper (He never did use them.) A most enjoyable day, though Graham seemed exhausted. I was concerned about his health, though he never complained.

I set off for Melbourne a day later than planned. Thomas clung to me and cried when he realized I was leaving, and I fought my own tears as I assured him of my return.

The next few days were a blend of work and play. I did a day's gardening at home, and had a restaurant meal with Ted, where we tried unsuccessfully to come to an amicable agreement over settlement. More pleasant meals were spent catching up with friends and former work colleagues.

Mum and I had a morning shopping and I did some gardening for her in the afternoon. Brenda joined us for dinner that night to celebrate her birthday prematurely, and we had a happy time. Bren is always good company, as she has Dad's quirky sense of humor.

Bob took me to the Mercy Hospital for my fifth chemo session and an overnight stay, and had me there at the required time of 10.30am. On inquiring what dose I would be given, they said it would be the same as the first time I was there. I reminded them that the dosage had been reduced, and the bags of drugs were re-ordered, with a long wait as a consequence. During the afternoon, the Professor who was head of the department came to see me.

He said that as my CA-125 had been consistently in the negative range (below 15) since my second treatment, there was no point in having further chemotherapy, as it had done its job. Yippee! He wanted to see me in three months time for a 'second-look laparotomy'. We'd see about that, I thought. *(See Appendix 4, 'Second Look Surgery')*

Chapter 3
Reclaiming my Life

New directions

On completion of my fifth and final dose of chemotherapy, I relaxed in a ward at the Mercy Hospital and slept until 5am; at which time the dreaded vomiting started again. An injection finally brought it under control. Bob picked me up mid morning and took me back to his home, where I slept in a drug infused haze most of the day and night.

The next day was Brenda's birthday, so I rang her to say "happy birthday", and Mum to tell her the good news about finishing chemotherapy. When I rang Katrina, she told me Rob's dad, Graham had undergone an emergency operation the day before for a tracheotomy, an opening into the windpipe to help him breathe, as his vocal cords were rigid. The family anxiously awaited the result of the biopsy.

Feeling a lot better the next morning, I was up well before Bob and gave the kitchen a good clean in appreciation of his care, and cooked him a hot breakfast when he finally emerged.

We then went shopping, and he helped me buy a second hand electric keyboard. I had decided to learn the piano as mental stimulation, as it had been brought home to me when I tried doing a crossword puzzle that my mental capacity was failing since my illness and treatment. Ted and I used to do them with ease over breakfast each morning, but I just looked at it and could barely start. Playing a musical instrument was something I had always yearned to do, but I hadn't even mastered the recorder at school. My aim was to learn some carols for Christmas and to that end Joan later lent me some lesson books, and Rob's mother Lesley, a piano teacher, gave me an introductory lesson.

After thanking Bob profusely for caring for me and being such a good and generous friend, I left to spend the weekend with Greg and Jane. A lovely couple of days together included a trip to the local nursery where Jane chose some roses, and we had fun planting them. Greg and Jane play in a mixed netball team, and I went along and cheered them to victory on the Sunday evening.

Monday, I headed back north, with a stop at Mum's on the way. On arrival, I was greeted by a very excited Thomas who was obviously glad to see me, and I happily took over his care from Rob, enabling him to get on with raking hay. Rob's new bale wrapper arrived later in the afternoon, and we were all impressed when he demonstrated his new 'toy'.

Tai Chi

Tai Chi classes commenced that evening. T'ai-chi Ch'uan, to use its full title, means 'supreme ultimate,' and was practised in China in the 14th century. It is a system of simple, slow, beautiful and graceful movements of the body, linked together in a dance-like formation, and often practiced in the open air. Although appearing deceptively simple, it is quite difficult to learn, and requires attendance at a number of weekly classes, taught by an experienced teacher. The short form consists of about 40 movements, while the long contains over 100, and can take more than half an hour to perform. Tai Chi is not used specifically for treating particular conditions, but held to be of value as a health promoting and life enhancing daily routine. Its effects help manage stress and tension, and diminish long-term muscular pain.

I had attended classes in Tai Chi at Healesville several years previously, and it had helped with the tension of living with Ted. This class was quite different, and I felt like a raw beginner again, but I decided to persevere.

It was good to be back home.

As part of the details of my financial settlement with Ted, I had to obtain current market valuations on my car and the land we owned in Londrigan, just out of Wangaratta. Ted and I had mortgaged our house to buy the five acres of land a couple of years earlier, and had planned building and moving there in the future, but the last twelve-month's events had put an end to those plans. I obtained the valuations on my next trip into Wangaratta and was mortified when my car was valued at only $500. I arranged for the land to be sold.

The next time I consulted the solicitor, she said she would only send one more letter to my husband's legal adviser before taking the case to court. I wrote Ted a letter containing some irrefutable facts, and asked him to try to see sense, and settle things intelligently.

Katrina, Thomas and Georgina (Rob's younger sister) and I, went to visit Graham in Albury Hospital. He was looking pretty good considering his ordeal, and could now talk a little. It was very upsetting for Georgina to see her father like that, so Thomas and I explored the hospital grounds to give them some time together.

Cancer Support Group

The Wangaratta Community Health Centre, in conjunction

with the oncology nurses, was running a Cancer Support Group, and I attended the first meeting. I was a little dubious about sitting around with a lot of sick people exchanging tales of gloom and doom, but it was nothing like that. Some participants had carers with them, a daughter, husband, or friend. Katrina would have liked to come with me, but five o'clock in the evening was not a convenient time for a young mother. Each participant had a different form of cancer and was having treatment according to the stage of their disease.

An excellent program of speakers and self-help programs was planned for the following weeks, and I came away in a more positive state of mind, following a light meal and a cuppa.

My latest CA-125 was 5.

Rob was up very early the next morning to take cattle to market. The full responsibility of the farm had fallen to him since his father's hospitalization, and there just weren't enough hours in the day, as silage and hay season was also in full swing. I was more than happy to help out where I could, and did the mowing and planted vegetable seedlings.

My back was troubling me somewhat the next morning, but I had promised Thomas an outing to the Wangaratta Show. He enjoyed seeing all the animals, and had a couple of rides and the usual junk food to eat, and thoroughly enjoyed the new experience. My back was really aching by the time we got back at lunchtime. I took a couple of strong analgesic tablets and lay down, but Lesley had asked me to accompany her to Albury Hospital to be with her when they spoke to the speech therapist; I'm not sure why, but I guess the moral support was helpful at such a stressful time. As it was, the therapist didn't show up, and I nearly fainted with the pain in my back and leg, which was very embarrassing, and it was an agonizing trip home. Graham was discharged soon after.

Retreating to bed, I only arose for trips to the bathroom for the next day and a half, tormented by some of the worst pain I had ever experienced. I was plunged once again into depression. What if my back never got better and I couldn't live a full and active life, a burden on Katrina and the rest of my family? I might as well be dead. A voice in my head reminded me that I was a humanBEING not a humanDOING, and for those who loved me, that was enough; what a difficult lesson for a person like me to learn. I prayed for relief and acceptance.

Katrina drove me to and from the chiropractor early the next week and my back had improved a little by the following day, enabling me to do some gentle walking. I met Graham at the letterbox and we had a short chat. There was no hint of the anxiety he must have felt as he awaited the biopsy result; he was such a stoic man.

Ted rang that afternoon to say the agent was coming to discuss auctioning the house, and he quibbled further over the settlement. Following a personal phone consultation with the agent, the date of the 29th of November was agreed upon for the auction. My final compromise over the financial settlement was that I'd agree to a 45/55 split, with the land as part of my settlement at current market value, and I finalised this with my solicitor.

Katrina came to me in tears later that day to tell me the biopsy had shown that Graham had cancer and was having his larynx removed the following Thursday week. My problems seemed so petty in comparison.

During the ensuing days, Katrina and Rob were kept busy on the farm cutting and bailing hay and working with the cattle, while I kept the home front going and looked after Thomas. I realised that I was retarding the rate of healing for my back, but considered I was not making it any worse as I rested as much as I could, and I was glad to be of some help.

Graham was to be admitted for his operation on the last week in October, so Katrina cooked him a special lunch before we drove him to Albury Hospital. I couldn't even start to imagine what it must have been like for him contemplating awaking after his operation unable to speak. The parts I had removed made very little impact on my day to day living. Katrina and I were subdued during our trip home, absorbed in our thoughts and sorrow over Graham's lot.

I developed some severe stomach pain later that afternoon, and vomited in the evening. By the following evening I had developed full-blown gastroenteritis.

It persisted into the next day, so I rang my physician for advice, and he said to go to Wangaratta Hospital by ambulance. On admission to emergency, an IV was inserted and X-rays and blood tests taken, then I was admitted to a ward until my discharge the following Sunday morning. Thomas was very excited to have me home again, but it was a terrible time of worry for both Katrina and Rob.

Knowing Ted's family were coming to Healesville for the weekend for a big working bee in the garden, I rang Ted on Sunday afternoon to see how it was going, and to tell him I'd been in hospital and wouldn't be down until the following week. The usual tale of woe was all I heard from Ted, though everybody had obviously been very kind and helpful, so I expressed my gratitude in a letter to them all.

Piano lessons

First piano lesson; wow! What a challenge. I couldn't even

read music, and my fingers wouldn't co-operate. At least the lesson books Joan had lent me made a little more sense now, and I practiced diligently a couple of times a day, and massaged my aching fingers in between.

With Graham in hospital, Lesley no longer looked after Thomas the mornings Katrina worked, so I had some early morning starts, but enjoyed the extra time with my darling grandson. The whole family was so stressed with the worry and extra work, that I became an integral part of keeping things going, and petty problems were put aside. One day, Katrina and I herded some bulls and steers into the yards on our own, and loaded them into the truck for market. We had just finished that when we received an SOS to chase some stray cattle out of Lesley's front garden. What a great team of cowgirls we were!

Having arrived at the stage where I couldn't bear to look in the mirror at my greying hair, I decided it was strong enough by now to tolerate dye, and the resulting effect had me feeling much better, and years younger. I found time to make the all-important Christmas puddings, and I also had a great time cultivating the vegetable garden into productivity, as Katrina had neither the time nor energy to do so.

On visiting Graham in hospital, we found him looking very ill and most frustrated at having to write notes and make gestures to be understood, now his larynx and vocal cords had been removed. I'll never complain about my form of cancer again, I thought. On another occasion, we took Graham's older sister Marjory to visit him. She has many health problems herself and Graham and she are very close. She became very upset, but was none-the-less glad to have seen him. It would be some time until he was able to eat and enjoy solid food again.

The first Saturday in November was Oxley craft market day, a must on our social calendar, and a diversion we felt we needed in the circumstances. There is always lots of lovely handcrafts available to buy as great Christmas presents, as well as local strawberries from which Katrina makes jam for her Melbourne friends, mountains of nuts, and a huge variety of herb plants, irresistible fudge, raffles, and kid's entertainment. We bought fresh bread for lunch from Milawa bakery on the way home, and felt in better spirits as a consequence of our outing.

The next day was the first open day at my Healesville home and only one inspection had taken place, which was disappointing.

The following Tuesday, I travelled down to Healesville to work for a couple of days sprucing up the house and garden, my last major effort before the auction. It was simpler to stay with Ted than at Mum's place, and after a cuppa on arrival, I set to thoroughly cleaning the kitchen. During the evening meal, Ted started arguing about money and settlement, ruining my appetite, so I escaped early to bed in the spare room.

House cleaning continued the next morning, and we gardened together all afternoon and were getting on quite amicably. Ted ruined the atmosphere later by launching into a tirade about refusing to stay in the house alone, and 'seeing me in court'. I had very little sleep that night. Following some washing and garden watering the next morning, I thankfully headed north again, leaving the house and garden looking a little more loved. Only one couple came through the house the next open day.

That evening was our cancer support group meeting, and we were led into a meditation by a natural therapist, which was exactly what I needed. I was so glad to be back in Byawatha again.

Graham was home at last and was looking very frail, but

he was mastering his electronic talking device quite well, making communication easier. He asked me if I'd go with him to check some cattle, which I was happy to do. Graham was teaching his dogs to respond to the blast of a whistle now that he could no longer call to them, and was starting to succeed. We saw a red-bellied black snake on the dam wall, a sure sign that summer had arrived.

I was persevering with my keyboard practice and slowly mastering some simple tunes, and was quite proud of myself, and enjoying Tai Chi, feeling the benefits of this ancient form of moving meditation.

An episode of blood in my urine and a bout of diarrhoea made me think I may have been over doing physical activities a bit, so I decided to slow down and not create more problems by becoming ill. A follow-up appointment at the Mercy Hospital was approaching, and I wanted to show my oncologist how well I had recovered and regained my health.

We had a naturopath speak at our support group meeting that week which was interesting and informative, and gave me an opportunity to share what I had learnt and implemented.

The All Clear

November 14th A nightmare trip south. I was on my way early, and half an hour down the freeway the rain started bucketing down. It cleared fifteen minutes later, but the wipers wouldn't turn off, and were scraping on the dry windscreen. When I stopped at Bonnie Doon, the half way mark of the journey, for a refreshment break, I rang Bob to see if there was anything I could do, but he was devoid of suggestions. The sound of the metal scraping on the dry screen due to the rubber blades shredding, nearly drove me crazy. On reaching Yarra Glen on the outskirts of suburbia, I had new rubbers fitted, but the wipers still wouldn't turn off, but at least it was raining again.

I arrived at Bob's by late morning feeling frazzled, and he drove me into Melbourne and the hospital for my appointment. My lovely gyn/oncologist said she could not see the advantage of me having the second-look laparotomy the Professor had suggested, as it was major surgery, and I was so well and showing no indication of recurrence. I was most relieved, and didn't tell her I was going to refuse surgery anyway. My ongoing instructions were to continue with the CA-125's three monthly. Samples of blood and urine were taken for testing before I left in a much lighter mood.

On inspecting and testing the wipers the next morning, Bob couldn't fault them! The favourite theory was that the motor driving them had shorted out with dampness.

Next on my agenda was a visit to my Healesville home to do some house and garden maintenance, calling in briefly to see Jane on the way.

After bringing in my baggage, I had lunch with Mum, then went over to see Ted. He lost his temper when I told him I'd be sleeping at Mum's, and started throwing and smashing things. I escaped into the garden and spent the time weeding and mulching. He eventually calmed down and said he would go to the movies with me as we had previously arranged. We saw *My Best Friend's Wedding*, a comedy that lightened the mood.

I continued with the house cleaning and gardening next morning, before returning to Mum's to prepare to attend a former nursing colleague's wedding. It was held in a large garden, with finger food to follow, and was a great chance to catch up with former nursing friends. One of them was in the process of treatment for Stage 1 ovarian cancer, and we exchanged experiences. She considered herself very lucky to have had the cancer detected and treated before it spread, but then I thought I was lucky too, for other reasons.

I would eventually go on to say that cancer was one of the best things to happen to me, as it gave me the chance to finally take charge of my life.

Shortly after returning to Byawatha was the much anticipated bus trip to Mt Macedon, and it was a long but most enjoyable day during which time Katrina's neighbour, Anna and I got to know each other better. I told her I would like to give something back to the community once I was feeling my old self again, and asked if she knew anywhere I could use my talents as a volunteer, and she made a few helpful suggestions.

On ringing the real estate agent the next day to discuss the auction, he said he knew of at least one person that would attend. I also rang the Mercy Hospital for the latest pathology results; My CA-125 was 9 and the urine test clear.

On the 22nd of November we celebrated Tom's second birthday, then it was on with the usual pre-Christmas preparations. A pleasant and unexpected surprise was a visit from my favorite Aunt and Uncle (Mum's younger brother). We enjoyed lunch together and then Noel and I exchanged anecdotes on piano lessons (he started formal lessons at 70 years of age). I demonstrated my limited skills, and he impressed me with his more advanced musical pieces.

I attended the last support group meeting for the year that evening, followed by a party to celebrate its success. We exchanged names and telephone numbers, and I remained in touch with a few of the girls. The best outcome for me from the group was meeting one of the other physicians practising in Wangaratta. He had been a guest speaker at one of the sessions, where I had asked several questions. This was a man with whom I thought I could communicate, so I asked my GP for the necessary referral. This proved to be a good move.

The auction, and the end of an era.

I travelled to Healesville early the day before the auction to meet with the agent for last minute instructions, and to do the final preparations to the house and garden.

Saturday 29th November. Auction day, timed for 3pm.

We were up early, but Ted was very tense and unable to concentrate on anything much. I filled vases with fresh flowers, dusted, vacuumed and mopped, and borrowed pot plants from Mum to adorn the verandah. It started raining at 2pm, just as Greg and Jane arrived to offer moral support. I brewed coffee and made scones as the agent had suggested, infusing the house with delicious aromas.

The auction was cancelled as only one person attended, and her offer was so ridiculously low, we declined it. That ended the day's activities, so the agent joined us for a feast of scones and coffee and a post-mortem discussion. When Ted and I were alone again, he fell apart, crying and feeling sick. I rang his family to explain the situation, and Anne suggested I retreat to Mum's for the night and not give him an audience to perform to. When he was in the toilet, I gathered my things and left, leaving him a note. I was pretty shaky and exhausted by then, so I had a long, relaxing bath and an early night.

After a refreshing night's sleep, I enjoyed a leisurely breakfast with Mum before venturing over to see Ted, finding him still miserable. On saying goodbye, he said he was so ill he didn't expect to see me again, but he'd try to hold on until the house sold! I hoped it would sell soon, for his sake, as he was taking the brunt of it all and was not coping well with the trauma.

I spent the rest of the day and night with Greg and Jane. Greg worked on my car while Jane and I did some gardening and walked the dogs. The following evening was spent with Bob, feasting on crayfish, potato salad, fresh asparagus and a bottle of wine while watching a video of *Madam Butterfly* on his wide screen TV; most enjoyable and relaxing. A few days later, he obtained tickets to take Isabel and I to a performance of *Messiah* at the State Theatre in Melbourne, on the 14th of December. I knew every word of Handel's glorious oratorio by heart, and had always wanted to attend a live performance, so I looked forward to the occasion with excited anticipation.

I was on the road to Healesville by nine o'clock the next morning and found that Ted was not home, so I loaded the box of Christmas decorations and a few more personal belongings into my car.

I later discovered that Ted had moved in with his younger daughter Debbie, and had the phone diverted there. Before returning to Byawatha, I visited the estate agent who told me he had conducted a good inspection of our house with a client the previous day. He explained that most properties sell within two or three weeks after auction, which was reassuring.

A solicitor's letter was awaiting me when I arrived back, stating that Ted would not agree to the 45/55 split I had proposed, and wanted 50%. I rang him and told him I'd never agree, even if the money were frozen until he died, and I planned a visit to my solicitor the following Thursday to make that official.

When I visited the solicitor as arranged, I directed

her to cease negotiations and to just draw up the papers as previously agreed and present them to Ted via his solicitor.

In the days that followed, backache and sciatica troubled me again, so I visited the chiropractor and took things a bit easier. I still managed to do some pre-Christmas cooking, making shortbread, mince tarts and truffles, both to eat and to give as gifts.

My back improved with a couple of day's moderation. One evening, Katrina, Rob and I had to make a mercy dash to one of the paddocks where silage bales were stored, as cattle had broken through the fence and were ripping open the wrapping. We all grabbed rolls of tape and patched what we could, but only managed to save a dozen or so of the 100 bales. Who'd be a farmer?

An offer had been made on our house, and negotiations were taking place. The buyer wanted a quick settlement, and offered $2,000 more if we'd settle before Christmas. Ted was all for getting it over and done with, and his family offered to move him out quickly.

I thought about it, and the pressure of doing all the packing and cleaning before Christmas, with nowhere to store everything, was more than I was willing to cope with. Ted was furious, and demanded I give him $1,000 of the forfeited money for settling in January. I refused.

The thought of having no home, no caravan, and no immediate prospects of accommodation in January depressed and worried me. Katrina and Rob had not been able to gain approval from the council for a granny flat on the farm, and the latest idea of building a big farm shed with a flat on the end of it for me to live in, was only in the planning stage.

Time to put worries aside and get on with the festive season.

I spent the next morning in the vegetable garden while Katrina baked. The contract of sale for the house in Healesville came in the mail, and I signed it and returned it by Express Post. The planning permit for the shed also came that day. The following day I signed the financial settlement papers at the solicitor's office, with the 45/55 split and the land as part of my share. With Ted's co-operation, all should come together, with settlement over on moving day. At last the saga of separation was coming to a successful end. What a relief.

Turning the corner

Why do I lose faith and give in to worry? Once again I had evidence of being looked after.

As I drove through El Dorado one day, I saw a house with a 'For Sale' sign. On inspection, I found it was a house I could easily imagine living in, situated less than five minutes drive from the cottage. On inquiring if it would be available to rent in four weeks time, I was overjoyed to be informed that the present tenants would be leaving the day before the settlement and moving-out day at Healesville was to take place.

The next task was to contact DSS and arrange for rent assistance to be added to my pension. I was aware that because the house was for sale I would only have a short-term lease, but that was an acceptable option considering my present situation; it looked like it was going to be a happy Christmas.

And it was.

Messiah was all I'd hoped for, with wonderful soloists, a glorious choir, and the chance to sing along with the Alleluia Chorus. In a Christmas card from Debbie, I received the news that her family was building a room on to their house for Ted, and a big workshop for him to potter in, which would surely give him security and keep him happily occupied.

Katrina and I cooked the first of two Christmas dinners on the Saturday before Christmas for all our family. Bren and her partner Kaye brought Mum up, and Greg and Jane, and Katrina and Greg's stepfamily also joined us. We served ham, duck and chicken cooked to perfection in the Weber, followed of course, by Christmas pudding. Greg and Jane stayed on after the others departed in the late afternoon, and we went to the local water hole for a swim so that Thomas could try out his new inflatable jacket, boat and ball. Katrina and I were alone with the remnants of the festivity by nine that evening, tired but satisfied.

Regrettably, the long day had proved too much for Mum, and she collapsed that night with dehydration. She was treated in the hospital emergency department and discharged into Brenda's care, nursing bruised ribs from her fall. She consequently rested quietly at home on Christmas day.

On the Sunday evening before Christmas, I attended a carol service at the lovely little Anglican Church in El Dorado.

When I got home, I found a very excited Thomas trying to coax his new kitten out from under the kitchen dresser. Katrina's cat was very put out about the kitten and spent a lot of time with me in the caravan, but I didn't mind at all, as I love cats.

We enjoyed a lovely Christmas day. Breakfast was pancakes and fresh raspberries, followed by an exchange of gifts. We then concentrated on lunch preparation, and set up the trestle on the verandah, which was still festooned with paper chains and tinsel from the previous weekend. Another slap-up feast with all the trimmings followed, this time for Rob's family. The greatest gift was having Graham join us; he had completed his last radium treatment on Christmas Eve. He and I toasted each other's remission, and future health and happiness.

Boxing Day was a relaxing one for everyone but Rob, as he was stripping the crop and worked from dawn to dusk every day until it was completed. The most strenuous thing I did was to remove the decorations from the verandah and ring Mum to see how she was. Her ribs were still sore, but she sounded much brighter.

As I was going to Venus Bay with Bob and his friends for the New Year, I packed up most of the things in the caravan, and stored them in Lesley and Graham's spare room. The short break away was the restful intermission I needed before packing up at Healesville and moving into my new home. As we toasted in the New Year at Venus Bay, I wondered how many more new years I would see in, and if I would make it to the twenty-first century.

1998 and the big move.

My New Year's resolution that year was to live my life, my way.

Returning to Byawatha on the second day of the New Year, I signed the lease for the house and spent my last night in the caravan before thoroughly cleaning it.

I travelled back to Healesville in early January, and met Ted at his solicitors to sign papers, then went to Mum's for lunch. Sorting and packing commenced that afternoon.

The next six days were spent working relentlessly. The removalists were horrified when they saw how far up the hill they would have to carry everything, and realized they'd under-quoted, but I had the original quote in writing, which I insisted they honour. They decided to spend the day packing the van, sleep in it, and then drive up north early the following morning. With his family's help, Ted had finished his packing and left the day before. He accepted the hug I offered before leaving.

Following a final, tearful circuit of my beautiful garden, I headed to my new home in El Dorado with a well-loaded vehicle, picking up the house keys and some food on the way through Wangaratta.

The removalists had already been there for an hour, and finding the house unlocked were half way through unloading. The house was easy to love, but the dry grass and half-dead garden was rather depressing. Once the removalists had departed, I returned to Wangaratta and purchased an evaporative cooler, and two goldfish for company.

Katrina and Thomas arrived as I was doing some unpacking, and Thomas was most impressed with my new home and wanted to cuddle the fish! I made a few phone calls to assure those interested that all had gone well, before falling exhausted into bed too tired to worry about being alone with strange noises.

Tuesday 13th January marked the first full day in my new home, eight months after the diagnosis of ovarian cancer, and what an eventful and life-changing time it had been.

Katrina and Thomas came around with some of his clothes and toys to put in the second bedroom. He had cried all the way home the day before, wanting to stay in my new house with me. Thomas tested the spare bed for size and comfort, and we talked about him staying overnight in the future, which satisfied him. Meanwhile, I spent every spare moment unpacking, creating the first home I had ever lived in on my own. That night, I discovered one of the many advantages of living alone, the free choice of TV programs!

Greg and Jane visited and spent a couple of days with

me. They replaced some of the things Ted had reclaimed, such as crockery and kitchen knives. Mum had already bought me some new saucepans. It was lovely having the family together again for a barbecue tea.

I decided to spend part of my settlement money (when it came through) on a much-needed car, and while I had Greg for his advice we prowled the Wangaratta car yards, but I ended up more confused than ever!

After Greg and Jane returned home, and on my next trip to Wangaratta, I called into the pet shop. I fell in love with a kitten, a beautiful silver-grey tabby I named Megan. She didn't take long to settle in and was wonderful company. She kept me smiling.

I was feeling very happy and at peace and sleeping better than I had in years.

Chapter 4

Full Remission, and more complementary therapies

Body and Mind

It was time to turn my back on the last five years. As always, my therapy was gardening, and I soon had a small vegetable garden under cultivation and started resurrecting the existing garden beds. This activity, along with mowing a large expanse of grass when it started growing again, helped build up my physical fitness. Time spent with Katrina and Thomas and a variety of houseguests from Melbourne held loneliness at bay, and I still helped out on the farm where I could.

The lease I signed was for a six-month period and it was always on my mind that the house was for sale and my tenure likely to be short lived. I approached Greg and Jane with the idea of them buying the house as an investment and using the rent as the loan repayment, but for various reasons it was not feasible.

The money from the financial settlement with Ted came through, which enabled me to replace my faithful old station wagon with a much younger Toyota Corolla. Thomas consequently christened me 'Ma Ma Blue Car' to distinguish me from his other grandmother.

My computer was up and running again and I continued with my writing once more. I joined U3A (University of the Third Age), which consisted of classes on various subjects for mature-aged people, without the pressure of exams. I attended classes in Music Appreciation, Philosophy and Australian Literature, which I found mentally stimulating and through which I met like-minded people my own age. It was then that I started a very important and close friendship with Pauline, also from El Dorado.

I also commenced group keyboard lessons through the Community Centre. My progress at home had ground to a halt, so this was just what I needed. It was a small class of mixed ages, but we were all at about the same stage of learning and encouraged each other. (The students gave a little recital at the end of the year and I was terribly nervous, but managed to get through my piece successfully).

A regular massage and monthly chiropractic adjustment kept my body toned, and during one of my massage sessions, I was asked if I'd like to see a visiting healer from the Philippines. He laid his hands over my back, abdomen and liver. The warmth and energy emanating from his hands was incredible and felt like electric vibrators. After saying, 'You will live many years and see your grandchildren grow,' he suggested I have apple cider vinegar and honey with my meals, and to 'speak to God regularly but briefly'. I left with a warm glow of happiness and well being.

Mum has been taking apple cider vinegar and honey for arthritis over many years, with very good results, and I had read a book of hers about the properties and uses of apple cider vinegar. As I recall, its benefits arise from the fact that it alkalizes the body, relieving inflammation and inhibiting the growth of bacteria and other foreign substances in the body. In the past I had used it in the water for my dairy goats on our hobby farm, as a successful preventative for mastitis.

I commenced having a teaspoon each of vinegar and honey, dissolved in warm water, with breakfast each day, an acquired, but not unpleasant taste.

My diet now consisted basically of fresh fruit and vegetables, organic where possible, whole grain bread and cereal (muesli), low-fat dairy products, fish and occasional chicken. I made fresh fruit and vegetable juice most days, and avoided caffeine. My beverages consisted of herb teas and roasted dandelion root 'coffee' (a liver tonic), and plenty of pure water. I continued with flaxseed oil and Percy's powder, and now the vinegar and honey mixture.

When I attended the Mercy Hospital in May, twelve months after my operation, I was given a clean bill of health as my cancer was in full remission. My CA-125 was 2.

Living alone had both advantages and disadvantages, including freedom to choose not just TV programs, but what and when I'd eat, though eating alone took a bit of getting used to. I solved this by having as many meals as possible outside on the verandah and my evening meal in front of TV. I relished mealtimes with guests.

Not sharing my bed and being able to read myself to sleep or have the radio on and spread myself out was something else I enjoyed, though Megan my kitten was welcome company on a cold night. Only having my own mess to clean up, which was minimal, and to be able to write uninterrupted were real bonuses.

I really missed the lack of a residential handy 'person'. To get anything fixed in the house, major or minor, entailed notifying the agent who contacted the owners (interstate), and then engaging the appropriate tradesperson. When the problem was a leaking gas regulator and leaky water tank, these delays were most inconvenient. I became increasingly proficient with a screwdriver, hammer and adjustable spanner.

It took me quite a while to adjust to being a tenant, having always owned my own home, and I was a bit paranoid about any accidental damage occurring leading to the loss of my bond money. I soon got over it, realizing that there was unlikely to be any more than normal wear and tear, which was acceptable. With the little jobs Greg and Bob did for me when they visited, I probably left the property in better condition than when I moved in.

There were times when I missed being a part of farm life but I still helped out at times, and now that I wasn't under the same roof as Rob, my relationship with him was more relaxed and comfortable, though never warm.

I kept in touch with Ted via occasional chatty letters, as phone calls only degenerated into bitter accusations from him about my supposed boyfriends. His mind was still torturing him and his lungs continued to deteriorate. In May, he had been admitted to hospital with a cyst on his lung, and I visited him there after returning Mum home following a short stay with me. He looked so sick and old; I could only feel compassion for him. He was discharged a few days later into his daughter Anne's care on a nebulizer, extra cortisone and antibiotics.

At about the same time, I saw some advertisements for 'Australia's Biggest Morning Tea', an annual fund raising event for cancer research for which individuals, groups or work places host morning tea, and those that attend make a donation. I rang for a hostess kit, after consultation with Katrina to see if she would assist me, and we each invited anyone we knew in the area. I also posted advertisements at the local store, the Community Health Centre in Wangaratta, and notified both the local paper and radio station. I was pretty nervous when the day came, as this was the biggest social event I had hosted for many years outside family gatherings. We had no idea how many would attend, so had baked more than enough for the nine that attended. We raised $140, an amazing amount as I had only expected the obligatory gold coin donation per person. It was well worth being so tired afterwards. We have made it a successful annual event ever since, in thanks for my recovery.

The Dream Holiday

Bob knew of my desire to see Central Australia and the far Northwest of Western Australia. It was a trip he had also dreamt of doing, so we discussed it and he said he would take me, so I started gathering information. But before we went on our trip together, I felt we had to define our relationship.

The last thing I ever wanted to do was hurt him, but I felt a strong need to be totally honest with Bob, and myself about my feelings. I felt that our friendship was very important and sincere, and was content with that. He wanted more. We tried it, but for me it didn't feel right. He was hurt and disappointed, and retreated to lick his wounds. Time healed and our friendship resumed, though never in quite the same way, as I felt guilty at having disappointed him by shattering his long held dream of us as a couple.

The trip eventuated in July. I insisted on single accommodation (at my expense), knowing that I would need some solitude to read, write, and meditate after spending all day and everyday with a busload of people. Bob was disappointed at first, but we both knew his snoring would disturb my sleep.

The trip on the Ghan from Adelaide to Alice Springs was wonderful. Seeing the vast expanse of desert by moonlight from my bunk, as we rushed through the night, was very special. I loved 'The Alice', and gained a whole new respect and understanding of the aborigines through various venues and speakers. Ayres Rock (Uluru) and The

Olgas (Kata Tjuta) were awe-inspiring. I found it strange to be seeing them in reality at last. It was almost like déjà vu, due to the wide media coverage they attracted.

We flew from there to Broome to join a camping tour to Darwin.

I had suggested an early morning flight from Broome to Cape Levique and over the horizontal waterfalls along the coast before joining the campers. I had seen it on a travel show and vowed that if I ever got to Western Australia I would seize the opportunity. It was breathtakingly beautiful flying over the islands and falls in the early morning light. Cape Levique is a pristine beach where we wandered for awhile before the return flight down the coast. Looking down, the water was so clear we could see sharks and stingrays swimming.

Camping was a challenge, as I had to erect and dismantle my own tent, but I soon mastered it. The bus was only half full, so we could spread ourselves out and each have two mattresses. They were a lovely band of fellow travellers. After setting up our tents and the camp kitchen each evening, we enjoyed Happy Hour while our meal was prepared. I can't remember ever having laughed as much as I did those evenings.

The scenery, needless to say, was stunning, and we indulged in it every way we could - walking, boating and flying - what a fabulous holiday destination. From Darwin we went to Kakadu for two days, and I was enchanted with the ancient landscape and myriad wildlife.

A virus infected everyone on the bus and I was the last to succumb, which made the flight home a struggle. I was going to bring Mum back home with me for a few days, but we postponed that idea, and somehow I got myself home, and went to bed for a few days.

Bob had been an ideal travelling companion, on the

holiday of a lifetime, and I will be eternally grateful to him for making that trip possible.

Heart and Soul

Relaxing meditation had become an integral part of my daily life; it kept me calm and centred. Books that I had been reading had caused me to wonder if I could take it further, so when Trisha, my favorite complementary therapist, invited me to attend a meditation group she was holding at her rooms, I took up the offer. The number of people attending varied, but there was a basic half dozen of us that did so regularly, and we formed a special bond of trust.

Trisha led the meditations and following the initial relaxation, she sometimes led us 'out of our bodies'. We all experienced this differently, and I found it most liberating and enlightening.

Although I had made good progress physically, I still felt emotionally traumatised and inhibited. Life with Ted had become a day-to-day battle for existence. The defensive wall I had built up around my feelings felt impenetrable, and I was like a prisoner, shutting others out and taking without being able to fully express the gratitude I felt. I had martyred myself in my marriage, which was destructive to us both. I was judgmental, embittered and angry, but in denial, as it all seemed too hard. At last I felt I was breaking through that barrier.

On one occasion, following our meditation, we each surrendered an item of jewellry and took a piece of someone else's, not knowing whose we had. Trisha asked us to hold it in our hand, close our eyes, and trust our intuition to give us a message about the owner. It was difficult to just let go and let something come, but we all gave ourselves to the experience and wrote down what had come to us. We then shared this, and in some cases the message had a profound meaning to that person. The participant who had drawn my watch had seen what looked like a black door with a bright light behind it.

It didn't mean much to me at the time, but I returned to Trisha for a kinergetics session and further explored what it could mean.

Kinesiology is the use of muscle response to identify areas of stress or dysfunction in the body's energy field. It can be used to identify and balance both physical problems that are causing dysfunction of tissues and organs, such as in food allergy, and also mental and emotional stresses that are blocking or sabotaging personal growth and affecting a person's ability to function effectively in the world.

As a diagnostic method, it was developed by an American osteopath early in the 1930s, and subsequently popularized by George Goodheart in the 1960s. The theory underlying Kinesiology is drawn from Chinese medicine, where it is believed that subtle changes to energy flow in the body occurs when an individual is in contact with a substance to which he or she is allergic. This can also take place if there is a mental 'allergy', or distressing emotion or memory associated with a particular person. In kinergetics, muscle testing is used to identify the area of stress, pain or imbalance, and also exactly where the correction is required. The only correction is Healing Energy, channeled through the hands. At a deeper level, it can be used to clear stresses in the subtle bodies. It was the latter application I was working through with Trisha.

She invited me to open the black door the participant holding my watch had seen, which she explained was the symbol of how I felt the need to control everything in my life, my inability to trust and have faith. I was living my life in fear, not faith.

I visualized opening the door, and behind it were a host of loving 'souls' radiating light and love. I let the light fill me, and felt the huge knot of tension and fear inside me beginning to soften. I wept with relief and joy. It took me some time of sitting quietly and having a cuppa before I could re-enter the reality of the day.

My daily meditation now took a different direction. After the relaxation, I was able to open myself to my guides and accept their love and guidance. I no longer felt so alone.

At about that time, I was reading *Conversations with God, Book 1,* by Neale Walsch, and came across this most appropriate passage.

> *'Every action taken by human beings is based on a thought of love or a thought of fear.*
> *Fear is the enemy which contracts, closes down, draws in, hides, hoards, harms.*
> *Love is the energy, which expands, opens up, sends out, reveals, shares, and heals.*
> *Fear wraps our bodies in clothing; love allows us to stand naked.*
> *Fear clings to and clutches all that we have; love gives all that we have away.*
> *Fear holds close; love holds dear.*
> *Fear grasps; love lets go.*
> *Fear rankles; love soothes.*
> *Fear attacks; love amends.'*

Ted rang me early one morning to tell me he was going to hospital again, he was depressed and was sure he was dying. I hadn't been able to completely turn my back on him and had even considered inviting him to stay with me between hospital stays. I didn't follow this through due to intervening circumstances, which I guess was just as well. I still lived in hope that he would find some peace in his life, and sent him love when I meditated.

I had several interesting experiences throughout 1998, which in hindsight were stepping stones in my spiritual development and enlightenment.

One Sunday in August, I went with some of the members of the meditation group to a seminar in Albury called 'Inner Healing'. It opened with a talk by an oncologist who specialized in palliative care. I was impressed by the peace I saw on his face and in his smile. I spoke to him briefly during the interval, and he encouraged me to keep following the path I was on. An Indian doctor then led a meditation, which she followed with a talk on meditation and its healing powers.

Later that same month, during a meditation session at Trisha's, I asked my guide if Katrina would have another baby. I then had the sensation of a baby lying in my arms, but I didn't tell Katrina of the experience at the time. A few weeks later when Katrina and I attended a workshop on 'Re-Set', an introduction to kinesiology, she told me she was pregnant again.

I was more excited by the prospect than they were at first, as Katrina had been constantly nauseated while pregnant with Thomas, and in a lot of pain with the extra weight, due to an injury to her back and pelvis, sustained when she was a teenager. They consoled themselves with the thought that it would be a girl. I had a feeling it mightn't be, and suggested to Katrina that she leave her mind open to the possibility of a boy, so that if it were, he wouldn't sense the disappointment they would obviously feel when he was born. She had an ultrasound at 18 weeks that looked as though she could be carrying a boy, and Katrina and Rob chose Alex as his name.

Another stepping-stone was when Trisha introduced the concept of Chakras, and we meditated on these several times. I purchased and read the book *Anatomy of the Spirit* by Caroline Myss, which I found very helpful, and remains by my bed for instant reference at times when I feel 'blocked'.

Chakra is a Sanskrit word meaning 'wheels' or 'circles of movement'. Chakras are spirals of concentrated life force, and are arrayed in a straight line in the front of the body, starting at the very base of the spine and extending to the top of the head.

The seven primary chakras are located as follows:

The first chakra is found at the base of the spine; the second a few inches below the navel; the third at the solar plexus; the fourth over the heart; the fifth over the throat; the sixth between the eyebrows; the seventh just above the crown of the head.

One of the functions of the chakras is to act as funnels for the life force. Each of us is continually bathed in an unlimited flow of electromagnetic energy, or the life force flow that sustains our lives. We breathe it in, receive it through the five senses, channel it through the field, and draw it into us through the seven chakras.

The chakras function on various levels; the physical level in relation to the organs of the body in their vicinity; and at emotional, psychological and spiritual levels as well.

Each chakra is the site of a specific consciousness, a realm that offers its own specific set of values. None of us has integrated all seven levels of consciousness into our being. The chakras therefore represent a kind of ladder of personal, psychological and spiritual evolution. Each of us is attempting to move into the next highest chakra; thus they describe in ascending order how we proceed from the very rudimentary consciousness to an ever-enlarging viewpoint on life and ourselves.

Following is a brief summary of the spiritual life lessons represented by the seven chakras.

The first chakra: lessons related to the material world.

The second chakra: lessons related to sexuality, work and physical desire.

The third chakra: lessons related to the ego, personality and self-esteem.

The fourth chakra: lessons related to love, forgiveness and compassion.

The fifth chakra: lessons related to will and self-expression.

The sixth chakra: lessons related to mind, intuition, insight and wisdom.

The seventh chakra: lessons related to spirituality.

Moving up the chakra ladder inevitably presents the greatest challenges life has to offer. Very often one or more of the chakras are blocked or partially closed, meaning that the life force is diminished to that part of the body, which can affect organs in the vicinity of that chakra, leading to dysfunction and/or disease.

This is a very basic and simplistic summary of the chakras and their function, but it may stimulate you to further reading on the subject.

Testing Times

In September my rental accommodation was sold, with settlement in early November. I was surprisingly calm at first, confident that everything would work out well and I would be looked after. I immediately started asking around about other houses to rent in El Dorado, and put a notice on the board at the local store. As the weeks passed, every house I looked at was not acceptable for one reason or another (derelict, not available soon enough, too expensive, etc), and my faith took a downhill slide. I became depressed and weepy, and couldn't sleep. Trisha gave me a lecture on being positive and trusting, but my old enemies of fear and the need to be in control won out most of the time.

As it seemed there was to be nothing suitable locally,

I started looking in Wangaratta, either something to rent or an investment property for Greg and Jane to buy then rent to me.

The houses for rent that I could afford were horrible, but I did find a lovely house for sale in a quiet back street. Greg and Jane came up to look at it and another house the agent showed them, but they weren't as enchanted as I was. Less than a week after that disappointment, a local lady, Lois, knocked on my door after having read my notice on the store's board. She asked if I would be interested in seeing the now empty granny flat on their property that they had erected for her late parents, and was now empty. On inspection, the size difference compared to the house I had been in was most apparent, but I did some measurements and mental furniture placement and decided most things would fit. Lois's husband Ivan was happy to continue mowing the lawn, and agreed to erect a small garden shed and a carport for me. I thankfully signed a 6-month lease from the 23rd of October. I had not only found a new home, but very special friends: I was being looked after.

Katrina's pregnancy was not going smoothly, so I was kept busy supporting and helping her as much as possible. My weekly meditation group continued, which included a new member, Doreen, with whom I got on very well.

I also attended a fascinating Intuitive Healing workshop one weekend in early October. We learnt to 'feel' each other's energy fields, and learnt about the qualities of different crystals, doing a couple of 'journeys' with a chosen crystal. I asked the leader of the workshop if he'd do a reading on my body (without giving him my medical history). He identified the missing parts of my anatomy and said my kidneys were okay, and he sensed the cysts on my liver. He said I needed to do more 'energy work', and still had to work on the cause of my cancer.

The second day of the course was intense and challenging, and I faced a lot of personal issues. I 'read' one of the other participants, but felt very inadequate.

On completion of the weekend we were expected to go into the community and charge to do readings on people, but that would be a long way in the future for me, if ever.

Another interesting experience was a session with a hypnotist, who led us in past-life regression. In one 'life' I was riding a donkey through the desert, which could explain my passion for donkeys and the determination to have them on our farm, but I wasn't fully convinced.

The rest of October was devoted to packing, cleaning and organizing the move, coupled with helping Katrina and attending my U3A and piano classes. Harvest was in full swing for Rob, and one day he was short of someone to drive the second tractor, which did the raking after he'd mowed, and the wrapping after he'd bailed. He asked if I'd give it a go. I had never driven a tractor before, but after a brief lesson, set off. My first rows were a bit erratic, but I soon got into the swing of it and became quite proud of my neatly raked rows, though I found the corners of the paddock tricky. Placing the wrapped bales in a straight line was also a challenge, but I met that eventually. I needed a soaking bath that night to get the crick out of my neck from looking over my shoulder all day. When I helped out again on another property a few days later, I went well all day. A couple of weeks later I repeated the process on my block, which Rob had sown rather than have it go to waste. He later sold that silage, which was a little bonus to my income.

Re-Settling

The move was spread over several days. Not everything had been unpacked from my previous move as I knew it was only a temporary home, so car loads of household items were transferred directly from the house to the unit, with Ivan helping out with plants and gardening tools in his trailer. Greg and Jane came up for the weekend move and helped with the heavy furniture items and unpacked boxes, and Katrina kept us well 'fed and watered'.

On my last day in the house, a journal entry says, 'I've been quite comfortable and happy here, but somehow it never really felt like my home. Maybe I won't get that feeling again, or even need it. As long as I'm happy, healthy and comfortable, that's all that matters, I guess.'

My cat Megan settled in quickly, and had Ivan's dogs under control in no time. I launched into the creation of new garden beds, with my landlord's blessing, and started a vegetable and herb garden.

I enjoyed making a home of the unit, and hung my pictures and unpacked and arranged my rather extensive owl collection. Mum came and stayed for a few days and enjoyed attending meditation with me. Brenda and Kaye also availed themselves of my hospitality, as did Bob and some other Melbourne friends.

Shortly after the move, I attended the Alternative Expo in Wangaratta, and sat in on a lecture about Reiki, something I hadn't come across before, and the concept appealed to me. I also had an astrology chart done, which indicated the future would not be all smooth sailing.

Life was busy, but good.

My faith was restored and I continued meditating. One morning Meg was on my knee when I journeyed to my place of peace, and I saw all the animals I had loved in my life. I hugged my donkeys and patted Wim, and cried with joy.

My CA-125 in November was 8.

November and December were full of the usual pre-Christmas preparations, with Thomas, now an active three year old, very excited. He was sitting on the kitchen bench helping me make chocolate truffles one afternoon in mid December, and accidentally knocked the big slab of marble that was there, on to my foot.

The result was a broken bone, which really slowed me down and altered some of our Christmas visiting arrangements. Luckily I had completed my shopping the day before, so everything worked out okay.

Christmas day, which was particularly hot, comprised a seafood lunch for Katrina, Rob, Thomas and me at my place, then the evening with Rob's family at his parents home. Katrina had driven me down to see Mum and Bren the previous weekend, and we met Greg and Jane at Bonnie Doon for a picnic.

1998 had been a very full and eventful year, and a cancer-free one, for which I was very grateful. It had included some new friendships, some of which I felt would get closer with time.

I had grown spiritually, and was feeling much more centred and at peace, and my brain had been stimulated with piano and U3A classes. The occasional yearning for a special, loving relationship with a man still visited me, but when I thought of sharing my bed and body, I wasn't so sure.

I now weighed 56kgs, which I wasn't too happy about, but I understood that the lack of stress and menopause were among the reasons for the weight gain. Anyway, Grandmas are meant to be cuddly!

In the back of my 1998 journal I had written a quote.

'People don't grow old – when they stop growing they become old.'

I hope I never stop growing.

Spreading my wings.

1999 was my 'golden year'. I was in full remission, felt happy, comfortable and secure living in the unit, and I even had access to a handyman again, what more could a girl want? My New Year resolution was to get fit, and help others.

When I rang Mum with New Year greetings, she sounded much brighter than she had been, and said how much she was enjoying a book I had lent her called *Ageless Body, Timeless Mind,* by Depak Chopra. I was to read a lot of very interesting and inspiring books during the next few years, including *The Celestine Prophecy,* by James Redfield, and *Conversations With God, books 1, 2 and 3, Friendship With God,* and *Communion With God,* all by Neale Walsch.

My daily routine would start with an early rise, then back to bed with a cuppa and a book before meditating, while the world was still at peace and just the birds were stirring. Meditation would commence with relaxation, and then quite often I would 'travel' to my favorite private place high on a rocky hill overlooking a ravine where all the animals I had loved were gathered. My guides would always be there. David, my higher self, was at my left shoulder, and other loving spirits would also be present. I didn't always know who they were, but sometimes I received a message from one or other of them.

One morning, Dad spoke to me. I always felt he was there, but hadn't particularly singled him out to speak to before. It was so real. I asked numerous questions about our relationship and my past and present life, and received loving and reassuring answers, some quite surprising. I told him how much Mum still missed him, and asked why he had left her when he did. The whole time I felt aglow with love; it was an incredibly profound experience.

When I 'came back', I wept for the loss of my father as I hadn't when he actually died.

Crying wasn't something I ever saw my parents do as I grew up, giving me the impression it wasn't acceptable behavior. When a favourite uncle and my dear grandfather died, I retreated from the house and family to cry, feeling weak and guilty succumbing to tears. Thank goodness I have now learnt to cry, though at times I still tend to be too self-controlled.

Although I cried over Dad, it was not just grief, it was also joy, knowing he was still so close and would be waiting for me on the other side. I rang Mum later in the day and told her the message Dad had sent to her and she was comforted by it, but still longed to communicate with him herself and wondered why she hadn't been able to.

In mid January, my friend Isabel who had lent me the caravan, suffered a marked deterioration in her health, and she was admitted to hospital. I visited her during my meditation to send her healing, and saw her surrounded by loving spirits. A few days later she lapsed into a coma and the family gathered around. The medical staff was still treating her, but to no avail, and it was decided to withdraw medication. Her husband Robert rang me several times needing an ear, and I was happy to lend it. He was naturally very distressed, as Isabel was having lucid moments and seemed disturbed, and he was in an emotional turmoil. I visited her in my meditation, and she told me she was worried about an unresolved problem with her sister. Both her parents (in spirit) and I tried assuring her that it was something her sister had to work out for herself, and that she would be all right. I took the risk and told Robert what I had done and what had been said. Not knowing anything about their family problems I wondered if he'd think I was some sort of interfering crackpot. Quite to the contrary, he convened a family conference and discussed what had happened, and it became a very positive experience for them.

They each went to visit Isabel and had a private conversation, saying what they needed to say, and said a loving goodbye. She died peacefully in early February.

Let's get Physical.

To improve my physical fitness, I accompanied Lois, my landlady, to 'Pryme Movers', a low-impact aerobics class run two mornings a week by the YMCA in Wangaratta. It was great fun, as well as a good, but not too exhausting workout, with a lovely bunch of fellow retirees. They were mostly women, one in her eighties.

I also joined the Warby Range Bushwalkers, another incredible group of energetic and enthusiastic older people. I was among the youngest in age in both groups, but certainly not in spirit. Walks were held twice a month, during which I enjoyed exploring the local and nearby landscape with this wonderful group of locals. I even led a couple of walks in Byawatha and El Dorado, to areas they had not as yet explored. My family bought me the required hiking boots for my birthday. They seemed so heavy and cumbersome when I first wore them, but I soon adapted. Carrying a backpack was something else I had to get used to, and it was sometimes the hardest part of a walk due to the arthritis in my neck, a legacy from a horse-riding accident many years previously.

Reiki

My friendship with Doreen, whom I had met at Trisha's meditation group, had deepened. In conversation one day, she asked me if I'd be interested in learning Reiki. She was a Reiki Master, and conducted training in her home when requested.

Among the many things Dad had said to me was that Doreen would be my teacher. It hadn't made a lot of sense at the time, but now it did.

Reiki is a Japanese word representing Universal Life Energy. REI describes the universal limitless aspect of the energy, and KI is the vital life force energy. Reiki accelerates the body's ability to heal ailments. It opens the mind and spirit to the cause of 'dis-ease' and pain, the necessity for taking responsibility for one's life, and the joys of balanced wellness. Of equal significance is the benefit that Reiki has of balancing at the mental, emotional and spiritual levels.

Masters teach their students the Usui System of Natural Healing in a two-day workshop. Students learn four attunements that align and open their energy centres to Reiki. They also learn the history of Reiki, the basic hand positions for treatment of themselves and others, and ways to use Reiki in their everyday lives. Class time is provided for students to begin practising Reiki on themselves and on the other students, under the caring supervision of the Reiki Master.

Reiki energy can be transmitted through many layers of clothing. A full treatment may take an hour and a half, and is very relaxing and meditative, as well as aiding healing. The transmission of the energy is stationary, unlike massage, and may be felt as gentle warmth, even strong heat or tingling. It distills a sense of peace and well-being.

The idea of Reiki had stayed in the back of my mind since attending a lecture the previous year, though I hadn't actively pursued it, but I now felt the time was right.

There was only one other student, so we had individual

and intense training. The first day was mostly theory, and covered a lot of what I had been doing by instinct during meditation. The second day was more practical, learning the hand positions, and how to 'tune in'.

We also went through several attunements. During one, my guide David left his position at my left shoulder and became integrated with my being, and I knew I'd never have to seek answers outside myself again; it was a deep and moving experience. We finished the day practising on each other. When the other student and Doreen gave me Reiki all over my body, I felt a great clearing, and my abdomen and legs felt better and lighter than they had in years. I was left in no doubt that this was what I wanted to be able to do for others.

Katrina was a very keen client, and felt great benefit from the sessions I gave her. Treating her also brought me in close contact with unborn Alex, contributing I believe, to the special affection we have for each other now.

Giving Reiki to myself also became part of my pre-rising routine, and I'm sure was of great benefit.

Back to Earth

I'm sure I don't need to tell anyone in the same situation that living on a pension is difficult. The residue of money from the financial settlement with Ted had been gobbled up with day-to-day living and moving expenses, and as the land still hadn't sold, I came up with a fund raising scheme. Making the family hot cross buns at Easter had become a tradition I started the year Katrina was born. They were more like rock cakes that first year, as I had lacked the patience to let them prove sufficiently. In fact, the abdominal pain I had after eating them was thought to be indigestion, so when I went into early labor to have Katrina prematurely, everyone was surprised!

My standard of bun making had improved greatly

over thirty years, I'm glad to say, so I decided to try and sell a few locally.

I composed and printed leaflets on my computer and did a local letterbox drop, and put a notice on the board at the local store. The response was incredible, to say the least. I had made 40 dozen buns by Easter, and was sick to death of them. Not having anticipated such a response, I hadn't bought the ingredients in bulk at a cheaper price, and had under-charged. There wasn't much profit in the enterprise considering the time and effort involved, but I did meet a lot more locals and received unsolicited orders for the following Easter.

Volunteering

In January, I read an article in the local Wangaratta paper about the Palliative Care Volunteer service. I had done Palliative Care training as a Registered Nurse in 1992, but retired from nursing before putting the training into practice. Being with dying patients and helping to ease their journey in any way I could, was an aspect of nursing that was special to me. Even when I cared for dying children during my training as a nurse, I experienced emotional pain, but there was also a special feeling present that's hard to explain.

The hardest but most worthwhile act I think I've ever undertaken was to voluntarily nurse the daughter of some friends of mine in their home, so that she could die in her own bed surrounded by the comfort of family and familiar things. Dying at home was not encouraged in the 1970s, but I knew their doctor from the Royal Children's Hospital, and he entrusted me with the drugs and the responsibility of when to give them. It was a terrifying responsibility, but a satisfying outcome for all concerned, and a life-long bond of friendship resulted from the experience.

I rang the number printed, and spoke at length to the

Palliative Care Volunteer's Co-ordinater. I agreed to attend a public meeting seeking more volunteers to be held in March. At the meeting, Doreen and other established volunteers attended to answer questions after the initial speaker had addressed those present. Being convinced this was my present calling, I came home with an application form and started the process of becoming a Palliative Care Volunteer. I passed the initial interview held before a panel of experts in the field, and commenced a nine-week training course in late April, not long before the birth of my next grandchild.

Katrina finished work in mid March, much to her physical relief but her employer's regret. It was thought that the baby was breech, but an ultrasound revealed it was in the correct position, however Katrina was carrying a big baby.

Her membranes ruptured at 1.15am on Friday the 4th of May, and I received an SOS call to stay with Thomas while Rob took Katrina to hospital. Her contractions started at 6.15am, and Alex was born at 9.20am, weighing a healthy 8lb 8ozs. Katrina was badly torn and had lots of stitches, but otherwise they were both well.

Rob came back to take Thomas to see his new brother, then when they returned, I visited. I had a lovely cuddle and changed Alex's nappy, then left Katrina to have some much-needed rest. In my journal I noted, 'I already love this beautiful child'.

And what a delight he has turned out to be. Thomas adored him from the start, and Alex settled down to a routine quickly, allowing Katrina to regain her strength and energy.

At that year's Biggest Morning Tea, my fellow trainees boosted numbers and Alex proved the centre of attention. Thomas played with other children attending with their mothers; it was an altogether successful day both socially and financially.

The Palliative Care training was both interesting and informative, and included visits to the two funeral parlours in Wangaratta. I found the 'back stage' tour fascinating. I had no idea there was such a range of coffins to choose from, with a variety of decorations, urns and associated paraphernalia. There was also a great range of pamphlets giving information for comfort and support to the bereaved, which I would be happy to refer future client's families to.

I was chatting to the director of the smaller of the two firms, and somehow got on to the subject of my miscarriages. He offered to try and trace the records to find out where their little bodies had been laid to rest, so I gave him all the relevant information I could think of, but to no avail. It seems they died just before all the present rules and regulations were put into place. He assured me they would have been properly buried, but the records just weren't available, and this gave me some peace of mind.

On completion of the training course, I had a further interview and was accepted as a volunteer. We had a celebratory lunch, and received our certificates, and very shortly afterwards I had my first client. He not only had cancer, but also advanced dementia. I couldn't communicate well with him, but was able to support his wife during the short time until his death, and for some months afterwards.

My second client was a lovely man, who died in peace at home surrounded by family, and I felt I had made a positive contribution. I had been reading *The Tibetan Book of Living and Dying,* by Sogyal Rinpoche during this time, and felt it had helped me in this work, as the basic philosophy of Buddhism is compassion.

My CA-125 in July was 8.

Also in July, I received the joyous news that Greg and Jane were expecting a baby the following March. Jane had an ultrasound at 18 weeks, and obtained a video recording of it to show us. They fast-forwarded the part where it was possible to determine the sex of the baby, as they wanted it to be their secret. Jane was well during her pregnancy, and kept her teaching job until the end of the year.

A couple of times during the latter part of that year, Greg had jobs in the Northeast, and it was practical for him to stay overnight with me. We had some great chats in the evenings, including how he felt about impending fatherhood. He was finding the prospect both exciting and daunting, as most trips into the unknown are.

During August, Trisha had a houseguest, Patricia, a friend of long standing on holiday from Queensland. She was a psychic, and used her skills and intuition to help people channel their energy positively. Patricia had been a great help to Katrina, so I decided to have a session with her. She said she was surprised at how 'advanced' I was and that she felt I had very little 'inconsequential karma' left, and no 'heavy energy' around me. She suggested I get in touch with Mother Earth and ask what I was meant to do next. Among other things, she perceived the closeness between Katrina and I, and most startling of all, said that Katrina's two children were the souls of the babies I had lost! I shared this perception with Katrina, and she was quite open and happy with the idea, but we have always kept it to ourselves. It didn't matter whether or not it was true, as I couldn't love them more than I do, but it was a comforting thought.

A real piano

That year, piano lessons were being held in the showroom of a local piano retailer. We were allowed to play whichever piano we chose, from the lovely old restored models, through to the modern uprights and the baby grand pianos. I tried them all and fell in love with the tone of a lovely old Wertheim, circa 1920. I was having trouble transposing from lessons on the piano to practice on the keyboard, each needing a different touch. During a visit to Bob's, I explained my problem and gathered the courage to ask him to lend me the money to buy the old piano, until I could pay him back when my land sold. He agreed, and wrote me a cheque, and I arranged the purchase on my way home. Re-arranging my furniture to make a place for the piano gave me even less space, but it was worth it. It took a while for my fingers to develop the extra strength required for the piano, but I was newly inspired, and my playing improved with conscientious practice. Thomas also enjoyed 'playing', as did my landlord's grandchildren when they visited.

Thomas was growing up so fast. He attended three-year-old kindergarten in El Dorado during the final term for that year, to prepare him for pre-school in Wangaratta in the New Year. It took a few sessions before he was happy for Katrina to leave him there, but his social skills improved, and he made new friends. Farm children are much more socially isolated from their peers than their city and suburban counterparts. They spend most of their time with one or other of their parents on and about the farm, or with extended family or neighbours, all mostly adults. I consider this a much healthier lifestyle physically and emotionally, but it does have its disadvantages.

Alex and I were also becoming well acquainted, as he was quite content to stay with me whenever Katrina needed a break. He seemed to accept me as a second mother, which gave me great joy.

At our Palliative Care Volunteers meeting in September,

the need for a regular newsletter was discussed. I offered to do it on the understanding that I would be learning as I went, as I had never done anything like that before. The first newsletter took me ages to lay out, but everyone was pleased with the result, and I went from strength to strength with subsequent issues. I introduced a thought for each month, along with the regular co-coordinator's message, summaries of the monthly meeting and any training sessions we had participated in, also inspirational texts I found or had been given, relevant to our work. Once I was into the swing of it, the newsletter took about four hours a month to do and was well received, an important communication tool for the volunteers and associated health carers.

My holiday, in October of '99, was to the Grampian Ranges in Western Victoria with the walking club. Accommodation was shared, with communal bathrooms and meals provided. It was basic, but clean and comfortable, and the food was great. Some of the walks were challenging and entailed ropes, but the scenery was fantastic and the wildflowers beautiful. I even had my first experience in a kayak on one of the lakes. My massage and Reiki skills were put to good use in the evenings to ease the aches of my fellow walkers. What a terrific group of people, and a very different type of holiday, during which I faced new challenges, and felt vitally alive. I had deliberately not disclosed the fact that I had cancer to anyone in this group, so I felt totally accepted for who I was as a person, and not as an invalid.

In November my CA-125 was 12, and Thomas turned four. My garden was flourishing, and I was asked to include it in an Open Garden Day in El Dorado the local Country Women's Association (CWA) was running. This was flattering and helped re-enforce my acceptance into the local community.

Christmas time again.

December was busy as usual, and began with my landlord Ivan's big 60th birthday party that I helped his wife Lois prepare and serve. I also hosted the Christmas barbecue for the Walking Club, which was very easy entertaining as everyone brought their own food and furniture and sat in groups around the garden. They also enjoyed the Christmas cake I provided.

I travelled to Mum's the week before Christmas and had time with her, Bren, and a variety of friends. It was Rob's sisters turn to host Christmas dinner and I contributed the pudding, all most enjoyable. Greg and Jane travelled up on Boxing Day and spent a couple of happy days with us.

There was endless talk of the possible catastrophes associated with Y2K in the build up to the New Millennium. I received instructions on how to set the clock on my computer to avoid any problems, but backed up all my important files on disk, just in case.

Pauline and I had grown closer during that year, and I joined her and her partner Fred for a picnic supper on Flat Rock - a scenic lookout in the El Dorado hills - to celebrate the coming of the New Year and the end of the last century. We shared a lovely bottle of '93 red with some gourmet nibbles, but retreated from the cold before the midnight hour. I watched the worldwide celebrations on TV until midnight, after which I lit my Peace Candle. The following is the story of the Peace Candle. I think it is worth sharing.

> 'Several years ago in London, a young man named Chris was diagnosed with leukemia. His

doctor informed him that his death was imminent and he could not expect to live longer than 3–6 months. He was advised to go home and make his arrangements.

Chris went home and completely fell apart for three weeks.

When all his anger was spent and he had no more tears left to cry, he began to feel urgency about making the very best use of the little time he had left. He thought about what the earth needed most and decided, as most people would, that it had to be 'World Peace', so he resolved to set about devoting himself whole-heartedly to this end.

Possessions no longer were a priority in Chris's life seeing as he would not need them after a couple of months. He sold what few he had and used the money to print leaflets aimed at raising people's awareness of the need for 'World Peace'. These he handed out to anyone who would take them on street corners all over London.

As the medical profession was unable to offer Chris any hope of recovery, he decided to take the matter into his own hands and at least aim for the highest possible quality of whatever life he had left. He saw an advertisement for Reiki and was attuned to levels one and two. This introduced him to an awareness of his spirituality, which he keenly pursued.

Three months passed by, then six, and he was still handing out leaflets.

Unfortunately though, his money was fast running out, so he used the last of his funds to start a small business for himself making candles and painting T–shirts with a 'World Peace' logo on them. These he sold on street corners to finance the printing of leaflets and to pay his rent and food.

One year passed by, then two, then three, and Chris was still handing out leaflets, and selling candles and T-shirts. He was at a social event one evening where he met the doctor who had diagnosed his illness three years earlier. The doctor was astounded to see Chris not only alive, but apparently quite well. He convinced Chris to be admitted into hospital for tests, and every one was amazed to find that all traces of leukemia had disappeared.

In 1997, the Dalai Lama was visiting London on a lecture tour. Chris went along to hear him speak, and afterwards went backstage. He explained his story to the Dalai Lama's helpers, and requested an audience with him for the following day. He agreed, so Chris arrived at his appointment with one of his hand made candles. He asked the Dalai Lama to light his candle and dedicate it to 'World Peace', with the idea that all candles lit from that one would carry with it his blessing and dedication.

Chris asked that all those candles be re-lit at midnight as we entered the year 2000, in the name of World Peace. Thousands of candles were lit from the original, and some were taken to at least five different countries. If this story and the flame were shared by all those who come in contact with it, by January in the year 2000, millions of people all over the world would be lighting their candles and directing their thoughts and energies to the concept of 'World Peace'.

Imagine if you will, the awesome power generated by such an act and the potential positive impact this could have on human kind. Perhaps you have said to yourself, "I am only one person, how can my meager efforts possibly make a difference to the scheme of things?" Here is your answer, positive changes on a global level need only require a small effort by individuals, and this is your chance to participate. ENJOY.'

Doreen, my Reiki master had given me one of the candles, so I purchased half a dozen more and lit them from mine, and printed out copies of the story before giving them to selected friends.

I also hoped that the peace I wished for the world in general would be reflected in my own life.

New Century, and more changes.

At 6.45am on January 1st 2000, the power went off; was the dreaded Y2K bug in action I wondered? Power was restored at 9.30am, so I checked if my computer was functional, and all was well.

My resolution for the New Year was not to put on any more weight (I was 60kgs), and my goals were to sell my land and to travel.

I always felt a bit flat in January. The Christmas excitement and socializing of December had been left behind, and most activities had been suspended. The chance to camp on Bogong High Plains with the walking group was an opportunity not to be missed.

I had never been above the snow line before, summer or winter. It was a bush camp with just a drop-toilet and a water tank, so we had to make do with a wash instead of a shower the two days we were there. I walked nearly 20 kms on the Saturday, and found it exhausting. The sight of some brumbies and the abundance of wildflowers made it worthwhile, but the bush and March flies were in plague proportions, nearly driving me crazy. We had a shorter walk to some cattlemen's huts on the Sunday, which was very interesting, but I was very glad to get home to a hot shower and a comfortable bed.

A camp at Mountain Creek the following month, at the foot of Mt Bogong - the highest mountain in Victoria - was much more enjoyable.

The rest of January consisted mainly of watering the garden and processing summer fruits into jams and preserves, something I have always enjoyed. Alex had been pulling himself up since before Christmas, and was obviously going to be an early walker, and following lessons, Thomas's swimming prowess had progressed to swimming under water with his eyes open, and diving. He still enjoyed a 'sleep-over' with me, with cuddles in bed in the mornings.

Greg and Jane were preparing a room for their baby, and I was attempting to make a quilt and matching soft toy. Handcrafts are not my strong point, and I found the whole exercise most frustrating, but the end product was colorful and functional; definitely a one-off.

My widowed friend, Robert became a grandfather again, a little dark-haired girl they named Isabel, and a space in his heart was filled.

The fees for piano lessons had escalated beyond my limited financial means, however my piano-playing uncle had sent me a lesson book of classics for beginners, so I set out to teach myself from that instead. In the meantime, the new program for the Community Centre was published and a local artist was offering drawing lessons at a reasonable cost, so I enrolled for those. I hadn't dabbled in art since my school days, but often wondered if I could learn to draw. The artist was an excellent teacher, and I thoroughly enjoyed the classes, and was quite proud of some of my efforts.

Maybe I could progress to illustrating the children's books I had written several years previously.

In early February, Thomas commenced pre-school, and Alex had his first 'swim' in the local water hole, which he didn't particularly enjoy.

Jane's baby was getting quite big by early March, so her doctor decided to induce the birth, which ended as an emergency Caesarian Section. Greg rang me at 10.15pm on the 5th of March to tell me about the birth of his new baby daughter, Samantha, who weighed in at 8lb 7ozs.

The following day I received an email photo of an exhausted-looking mother and sleeping child, and the following day, more photos and some sounds; the wonder of modern electronics! It was almost as good as being there.

Greg was an extremely proud father, and was more involved and confident than he had expected to be. He soon took over the daily bath routine, and together they were a very happy little family.

I travelled down to visit and deliver the quilt and other gifts when Jane was settled back home. Samantha was a beautiful baby, and I enjoyed lots of cuddles. Greg and Jane took her to show Mum, and she was thrilled to have a great grand daughter at last.

On The Move Again

Shortly after the joyous birth of my grand daughter, Lois came over to tell me they would not be renewing my lease in April. Their daughter and her two children needed a place to live, and although I understood the situation and said I would do the same in her position, it still came as a great blow. I felt so at home and secure there and really wondered why I had to be uprooted again.

I had a big cry and became depressed for a short while

then picked myself up and started house hunting. The locals were most helpful with suggestions, but I wasn't having much luck finding anywhere suitable. Units I could afford in Wangaratta were depressingly basic, and wouldn't allow a cat. Finally, Rob's dad Graham told me about an empty house he knew of on the outskirts of El Dorado, in the middle of a 1,000-acre grazing property. I met the owner and looked over it. It was larger than I needed, but I really liked it, as did Katrina and Thomas.

It was white weatherboard, with verandahs front and side. The original back verandah had been enclosed, and made a great space for children to play in, or for entertaining. I loved the big family kitchen, the heart of a country house, and I could envisage my piano in the cosy lounge room, with its French doors opening onto the verandah. The rest of the house comprised three large bedrooms, a lovely bathroom, and a formal dining room.

The laundry and toilet were off the back verandah. The high ceilings with their decorative roses and cornices added to its charm. Built in the 1920s, it was showing its age a little, but that added to its character.

The rent was $30 a week more than the unit, which was really going to strain the budget, but I didn't have any other choice in the end, and decided to take it.

During the following few weeks I fitted packing and extra house cleaning into my routine, and converted my vegetable patch back into lawn and generally trimmed and tidied the garden. Thomas became very competent with the secateurs, and Alex took his first two steps in the garden. His happy smiling face with its halo of white-blonde hair as he staggered towards me was a joyous moment. Wherever he went he smiled and laughed, and the glummest person couldn't help smiling in return. It was a real tonic to have him in the trolley at the supermarket as he spread his sunshine.

Moving day approached and I went over to check out my new home, called 'Pleasant View'. In the six months it had been vacant, the termites and mice had invaded and made a lot of mess. The owner arranged for it to be sprayed, which entailed drilling holes in the concrete verandah, and lifting carpet and floorboards in the house, it looked like a bomb had hit it! I asked if he'd have it professionally cleaned before I moved in, which he agreed to do. It was not to my standard, but better than it had been, but I still had to arrange for an electrician to replace power points in the kitchen that had been shorted out because of the termites and possums. The shower rose was blocked, the phone hadn't been connected, taps dripped, doors jammed, the oven door was unsealed. All these and other minor problems were eventually fixed, but it was a very stressful time.

A kindly neighbour in El Dorado who used to work as a furniture removalist, offered to use his piano trolley for moving the piano, my greatest concern, and said he'd be happy to drive the truck if I hired one for the move. He, Ivan, Rob, Katrina and I worked like slaves on moving day, and had most of the furniture and boxes transferred by lunchtime. Katrina prepared us a delicious lunch before I finished cleaning the unit.

I kept Megan in the house with me the first night, and after she was replete with mice, she slept on my bed. The fumes from the termite spray were still in the house, which gave me a thumping headache by morning.

Rob was on night shift for Katrina's birthday, which was two days after the move, so we celebrated in my new home, and she and the boys stayed overnight.

Thomas loved the house, so much room to run and play, and one of the bedrooms had been put aside as their playroom. We had great fun exploring the farm sheds and finding 'treasures'. There was also a tennis court on the property, so Katrina hunted out some old tennis rackets and we had a hit. I had the use of a garage and a storage shed, and I obtained permission to keep chooks in the substantial poultry shed. Tom's pet chicken, 'Little Foot', was the first resident after she had grown up, and some neighbours donated a few more hens they no longer wanted, so I was soon enjoying fresh eggs.

The garden had grown wild, but I already had plans to resurrect it. It turned out to be a much bigger and harder task than I had anticipated, as the huge established trees had invaded and choked all the garden beds with their roots, but I persevered. There were some beautiful old roses, which I pruned and fed back to their former glory, and some lovely flag irises and canna lilies I spread around. Four huge elms shaded the back of the house, but they had suckered everywhere and blocked the drains with their roots.

They also provided mountains of leaves in autumn, which I used to mulch the garden, along with the sheep manure I raked out from under the property's shearing shed.

It took me eighteen months and many backaches until I completed the task and was happy with the result. (I opened the garden to the public in October 2001 as part of a fund-raiser for the local school, which Tom by then attended.)

My friend Joan came and stayed not long after I moved in and loved the place, as did Mum and Brenda when they paid a visit. Greg, Jane and Samantha spent the Easter break with me and made the most of the tennis court while I happily spent precious time with the baby.

In May, we celebrated Alex's 1st birthday, and my 56th, three years after my operation. The back verandah was the perfect space for the Biggest Morning Tea, and more people than ever attended, some of them enjoying a game of tennis.

Sadly, Graham's cancer had returned as spots on his lungs, and he commenced a heavy regime of chemotherapy. He was never a big man, and we were saddened to see him so thin and pale. Katrina and I tempted him with special food, and I gave him Reiki. Knowing I had also experienced chemotherapy seemed to make him comfortable being with me. My own blood tests had been normal for so long now and I was only having them every six months, so I was quietly confident I was cured, but Graham's relapse made me realize I couldn't afford to be complacent.

A change of view

I settled down to a routine in my new home, the days and weeks blending into each other with the regular sameness of housework, gardening, Palliative Care clients, meetings and newsletters, and piano practice.

I still had time with the boys; these were my most precious moments, savouring their unconditional love, their honesty, and sharing their wonder as they discovered the world around them. Except for the days we spent gathering firewood, I had very little involvement with the farm, which I missed.

It was incredibly quiet in my big house. I would lie awake at night in the pitch dark and not hear a single sound. I could have been alone on a desert island.

When did my life lose meaning and start feeling like I was just filling in time?

In June, an entry in my journal says, 'I don't know why I keep this diary of my boring life', and again, 'Feeling depressed – why? Maybe it's because I don't have a dream to work towards, and anyone to share it with, one to one.'

I was certainly never bored, and had some great friends and interesting occupations, and did some worthwhile things, but I always came home to an empty house. No one to greet me with a warm hello and a cuppa, and no one to share thoughts and feelings about the past day with. I had never got used to eating alone.

What of Ted and Bob? Ted had admitted himself into a hostel where I visited from time to time. He sent me some stamps in the hope I would resume writing to him. I did so intermittently, sharing the highlights of my life including my excursions with the walking club. He rang me some months later very agitated, and told me not to write again telling him about holidays with my boyfriends, and accusing me of putting him in the hostel. I hung up on him. A couple of weeks later I received a letter from him stating that he knew I never loved him, and the separation had caused his illness. I didn't bother replying.

As for Bob and I, our friendship continued, but on a much cooler level.

He bought himself a campervan and took off on extended holidays, calling in to stay overnight if he was passing my way. We chatted and shared outings, but it was never as comfortable as it used to be, always that disappointed expectation of his hanging over us.

Was I destined to follow in the footsteps of my grandmother, mother and sister and live for years on my own, alone and independent, living my life on the fringe of other people's, gaining succor from their friendship and love? Was I an emotional cripple, unable to give myself totally to another, and love and be loved unconditionally?

My CA-125 of 33 in August would show that the remnants of cancer in my body became active again at the time my thoughts changed from positive to negative. A coincidence? I don't think so.

I took these questions and feelings to a kinergetics session with Trisha. She suggested that when I meditate, I visualize my spirit as a candle flame, now burning dully, and bring it back to when it was bright.

I was able to do this one morning, and went on to visualize myself walking along a beach. I came upon a row of doors. I chose one at the left-hand end that seemed to lure me with its brightness. It opened before me, and I was in a town setting of the 19th century. It was an affluent area, and I could feel myself dressed in a resisting corset or bodice of some kind, and a long skirt, bonnet, gloves and carrying a reticule. I walked along and thought of my children, and a nanny brought them to me and they ran into my arms. It was Katrina and Greg, but they were dressed appropriately for the era, and were named Mary and Alfred; I was Evelyn. We went to the park, and I sat on a bench and watched them play. I was thinking lovingly and happily of my husband Robert, a doctor.

The children and I walked a short way home to an elegant house with steps up to the front door. Martha, the housekeeper, made us tea. Robert came home and we embraced. I was very happy. He treated me as an equal, and told me of his day. I knew I worked as a volunteer at the hospital, and brought great comfort to the sick as we worked together there.

Next - it was many years later - Robert was dead. I was lying in a big bed, dying and I was aware of a mass in my abdomen. My children and grandchildren and old Martha surrounded me, and I bade them a fond goodbye. Robert was standing at the end of the bed waiting for me with open arms. I gladly left my body and went to him and we were reunited, and I felt complete joy.

When I returned to the present, I wrote all this in my journal, but was left with the questions. 'Why haven't

I met him again in this lifetime? Will I? Where is he? I believe we will be together again some time, as we are obviously perfect together, and God loves perfection, love and happiness.'

I vowed to keep my flame as bright as it was then, in the hope that he will see it and be attracted back to me.

Trisha also suggested I read Depak Chopra's *The Path to Love*, and this passage held particular significance for me.

> *'Self love grows when you refuse to follow the impulse of anger and fear; trust that the universe is on your side; form your desires from the heart and watch the higher self carry them out; believe that you are enough in and of yourself; heed the tenderness and sweetness of your love for others; put your attention on positive energies in every situation; honor your own needs without having to seek outside approval; and cultivate the peace of inner silence.'*

In July, I saw a program on TV called *Somebody's Mother*, made by a journalist whose mother had died of ovarian cancer. At the end, it gave the web site address of OVCA Australia. I was not connected to the Internet at that time, so I asked Katrina if I could access the site on their computer. On doing so, I discovered they had a 'buddy' support system, so I entered my details and took note of the email addresses of some women in a similar position to me, with the aim of contacting them.

The ones I contacted didn't reply, but I received quite a few inquiries from within Australia, the USA, and elsewhere. Some were short-term exchanges, but I built up relationships with several others, for various lengths of time. We exchanged experiences and feelings, and I was often asked about the complementary therapies I had used, and the books I had found helpful. I am still in touch with a buddy in New York, and I became very close to one in Townsville, Queensland. She sent me this lovely piece on friendship.

'People come into your life for a **reason**, a **season** or a **lifetime**. When you figure out which one it is, you will know what to do for each person.

When someone is in your life for a **reason**, it is usually to meet a need you have expressed. They have come to assist you through a difficulty, to provide you with guidance and support, to aid you physically, emotionally, or spiritually.

They may seem like a Godsend, and they are! They are there for the reason you need them to be. Then, without any wrongdoing on your part, or at an inconvenient time, this person will say or do something to bring the relationship to an end. Sometimes they die. Sometimes they walk away.

Sometimes they act up and force you to take a stand. What we must realize is that our need has been met, our desire fulfilled, their work is done. The prayer you sent up has been answered, and now it is time to move on.

When people come into your life for a **season**, it is because your turn has come to share, grow, or learn. They bring you an experience of peace, or make you laugh. They may teach you something you have never done. They usually give you an unbelievable amount of joy. Believe it, it is real; but only for a season.

Lifetime relationships teach you lifetime lessons; things you must build upon in order to have a solid emotional foundation. Your job is to accept the lesson, love the person, and put what you have learned to use in all other relationships and areas of your life.'

It was great to be able to communicate with women who understood how I was feeling, and I was glad to be able to share the knowledge I had.

Life goes on

My current Palliative Care client was a sweet little lady with chronic lung disease. She and her husband were well advanced in years, and he was finding it very difficult to care for her adequately at home. They were absolutely devoted to each other, and the thought of being parted was terrible, but in the end it was unavoidable. The husband started writing notes about his life history for the family, and I offered to type them up for him. He had had minimal schooling, and was finding it hard going, but it kept him occupied and to an extent, took his mind off his loneliness.

I found it a great privilege working with this lovely, gentle man. He had grown up on a farm in Byawatha, so I could relate to the areas he was writing about. I kept to his own words as much as possible, and always checked back with him after each section.

This went on for several months, and he was pleased with the end result, and I felt it was one of the most worthwhile things I had ever done with my writing.

The whole of Australia was gripped by Olympic fever that year, and we had reason to be proud of both the organizers and the athletes, as well as the volunteers, including Rob's mum, Lesley, who helped make the overseas visitors welcome. The Olympic flame came through Wangaratta, and Katrina, the boys and I, joined in the festivities. I maneuvered Thomas to a front row position as ex-Olympian and local boy Dean Woods carried the flame aloft as he rode his bike towards the podium. Thomas was very excited and most impressed.

During that winter, I burnt the back of my hand putting wood on the fire, and despite due care, it became chronically infected into my knuckle. This put an end to piano practice for quite some time, and I never really got back into it. After two courses of antibiotics, my knuckle was still sore, swollen and aching. It was really getting me down. During meditation one morning, I asked my guides some questions.

'Why won't my hand get better?'

'It is to slow you down, stop you doing too much, to protect you.'

'How long?'

'As long as necessary'

"Will I play the piano again?'

'Try. You will be able to do all that is necessary.'

'What about my relationship with Bob?'

'You will both get the amount of love you need without being dependent. We don't want to see you making the same mistakes again.'

Over the Melbourne Cup long weekend in November, Greg, Jane and Samantha came to stay. Katrina and I put on a surprise 30th birthday party for Greg, which he enjoyed, and much tennis was played. Sam was pulling herself up on the furniture, and all three cousins shared a bath, with much laughter and splashing. Such happy memories.

A couple of months earlier I had got tired of penny-pinching, and decided it was time to urge the real estate agent into action to sell my land. I wrote an advertisement, and asked them to make an effort. In late November, my land sold, with settlement in late February. HOORAY!

I celebrated my new financial freedom with a weekend

away with Joan and my life-long friend, Margot. We spent it at her holiday house in Anglesea on the south coast of Victoria, an easy drive from Melbourne. The following weekend I camped on Mt Buffalo with the walking group. This was also the weekend Greg and Jane moved house.

Thomas had turned five and celebrated with friends from pre-school at his first real party, just prior to Orientation Day at the small local school he would be attending the following year. Katrina purchased his uniform, and he tried it on when he got home. He didn't want to take it off, so ended up sleeping in it, clutching his new school bag. Alex had stayed with me for his afternoon nap while Katrina and Tom attended school. When he awoke, he snuggled up on my knee until he was fully awake, and spontaneously gave me a big, wet kiss; I was over the moon with joy.

We Palliative Care Volunteers celebrated the end of a year's work with an evening cruise on Lake Mullwala, out of Yarrawonga, and it was most enjoyable. Once again I hosted the walking club Christmas get together. Among a variety of other end of year events was Tom's pre-school concert. He played the part of an angel, a very fidgety one, in the nativity play, and really got involved in the singing. He had the job of speechmaker on behalf of the children, and thanked the parents 'from' coming along. We were so proud of him.

Among my Christmas cards was one from Ted addressed to 'Marion and your boyfriends'; poor tormented man.

Our family gathered in Greg and Jane's new home on Christmas Eve. I picked up Mum, and Katrina and the boys came down (Rob was too busy harvesting), and Bren and Kaye joined us. The little cousins had a wonderful time tearing into their gifts after we'd shared a delicious dinner and my pudding. Back home, my New Years Eve was spent minding the boys while Katrina and Rob attended a neighborhood party.

My New Year resolutions were to stay healthy and have a reason for being so, to continue to grow spiritually, and to make a difference in a positive way to others. I also wanted to resume the piano and continue to learn and improve, and to use my money wisely.

Just prior to Christmas, one of my OVCA buddies, K. who had been living in the Philippines, decided to move to nearby Bright to be with her son. We arranged to meet in Wangaratta for a chat and we got on really well. It was great to have actual physical contact with a buddy. Her CA-125 had started to climb again after being in remission for some time, and she had to make decisions about ongoing treatment.

She ultimately decided against further chemotherapy treatment, and had some positive response from ozone therapy in Melbourne. She travelled to Queensland the following year to pursue a variety of alternative therapies, including having her amalgam fillings removed and replaced.

On the other hand, my buddy in Townsville, J. was at a similar stage of her disease and decided to avail herself of anything and everything the medical profession could offer, and had operations and various chemotherapy drug combinations.

I continued to send them both love and healing when I meditated.

CHAPTER 5

'I'm Back' - CA -125 starts rising again

2001

Ever had one of those weeks when everything goes wrong? I had one the first week of January 2001.

It started with a minor irritation when I went shopping to stock up after the holiday break. Firstly, my EFTPOS card wouldn't work, and I had to walk all the way to the bank, get out cash, and order a new card. We were in the middle of a heat wave, so I was not impressed.

Then the news came that Bob had been having angina attacks (again), and had decided to see the doctor, who ordered stress tests for the following week. I urged him, as I had been doing for years, to improve his diet and cut down on his drinking, but it fell on deaf ears as usual. He only managed the second level of the test, and was ordered an angiogram for the following week.

I had my routine blood test, and it was rather a shock when my GP rang me with the result; my CA-125 was 170, up from 33 six months previously. She ordered a range of blood tests and a CT scan. While I was at the hospital having the scan, Graham was being operated on for a strangulated hernia.

To round off the week, my VCR chewed up a tape and had to be taken in for repair, my printer went on strike, and the manuscript of my children's stories was returned from the publisher unread, 'too many submissions lately.'

Surely things could only get better after a week like that!

I decided it was time to see Trisha for a massage and intuitive screening. She decided my right side was most affected because I was denying my 'masculine side'. I had been having a lot of pain in my right shoulder, and a persistent niggle in the lower right side of my abdomen lately, which I suspected could be related to the cancer. We went on to explore relationships with important males in my life, from my father onwards. With the help of some kinergetics muscle testing, it was decided I'd try a Radical Forgiveness exercise, focusing on my first husband. I imagined him sitting in a chair opposite me and with Trisha's guidance, asked him relevant questions, and imagined what answers he'd give.

The process of Radical Forgiveness gives you the opportunity to resolve relationships you are reacting to and judging. We often react to the people who are most like us, for they show us the parts of ourselves we don't like. Any situation you find challenging is showing up your beliefs about yourself, and providing an opportunity for positive insight and experience.

Everyday, life feeds back to us our interpretation of reality. If you don't like that reality, radical forgiveness gives you the opportunity to change yourself and that life script.

It was emotionally draining, but most therapeutic, and I noticed over the next few days that the abdominal pain had disappeared.

My CT scan was clear except for the benign lesions I knew were on the underside of my liver, so more blood tests and an ultrasound were ordered.

Bob rang and suggested he stay with me for a month

so I could prepare him healthy food and encourage him to 'dry out'. I felt I had enough problems of my own and was less than polite about the idea, and had to ring him back the following day to apologize. His angiogram revealed three blocked arteries, and he went on the waiting list for surgery.

I had the ultrasound and awaited the results.

I awoke in the small hours of the following morning and started thinking about all the good things that had occurred in the past three years. Two more grandchildren, some good new friends, especially Pauline, Doreen, Lois and Ivan, and reconnection with important old friends, namely Margot and Joan. I'd had some great walks in Northeast Victoria and the Grampians, created some gardens, was able to help and support people through Palliative Care and OVCA buddies, and saw Greg and Jane settled into their new home.

Then I thought of what regrets I might have if my end was near. Not having my children's books published was my first thought, so I decided to investigate self-publishing. I would also work on seeing the Great Barrier Reef, and flying over Antarctica.

I had an appointment with my physician to discuss the test results, which were inconclusive, and all the blood tests were normal. He wanted me to see an oncologist back at the Mercy Hospital, so I made an outpatient appointment for early February.

He also gave me some information he had found on the net about the CA-125 blood test. It was most interesting, and I was encouraged by the statistic that if it drops after three doses of chemotherapy, as mine had, the prognosis was good.

Meantime, I filled my days making vast quantities of tomato sauce and relish, and endlessly watering the garden. Thank goodness we could retreat to the local water hole for a regular cooling swim. Both the boys were real little water babies by now.

On Australia Day, we had a huge storm and 36mm of rain, some of which entered my house, but was easily cleaned up. We were then back to our more normal summer weather of clear hot days and cooler nights, thank goodness.

Bob sent me an email saying he thought our relationship might be one of the great 'could have beens' that never got past the wishing stage. We had a long, honest talk on the phone, and got our relationship back on a comfortable footing.

Pauline and I discussed going to Lord Howe Island - situated on the tip of the Barrier Reef - during the coming winter, and obtained some information from a travel agent.

Thomas commenced school. His parents accompanied him the first day, and he was quite happy when they left. On his second morning he caught the school bus, which picked him up at the front gate, and he quickly made friends with the driver and the other children. I guessed I wouldn't be seeing as much of him from then on.

Biting the bullet.

I took the train into Melbourne for my outpatient's appointment. My previous oncologists no longer worked there, so a very earnest young man I hadn't met before saw me. He examined me thoroughly after reading my medical history, and the letter and test results I had brought with me. He disappeared for some time to consult his superior, whom I never saw, then returned to inform me that I needed to repeat the chemotherapy I had undertaken previously, as soon as possible. I was then sent to pathology for another CA-125, which took two technicians three attempts to obtain. I was feeling very emotionally traumatised when I met Bob in the cafeteria for a drink, as previously arranged. We had a stroll in the nearby park before going our separate ways.

I had three hours on the train to brood over the day's events. It wasn't so much the advice to have more chemo that upset me, I could have guessed that, but the way it was presented. Unlike my previous oncologist, this young man didn't seem to take my feelings into consideration.

I wasn't asked how I felt about it, or if there were any questions I wanted to ask. Where was my oncologist when I needed her?

I was feeling really flat by the time I got home. I decided a couple of days later to seek her out, and after some detective work, rang for an appointment to see her privately, no matter the cost.

That day, the money from my land sale was deposited in my bank account. The first thing I did was to write out cheques to those family members and friends who had loaned me money. I also supported some of my favourite charities, and bought myself a much-needed freezer for my surplus summer produce.

The next time I spoke to Greg to catch up on news, he told me he'd had a medical checkup for insurance, and his blood pressure was far higher than it should be. I read him the riot act about diet and exercise, and cited Bob as an example of what could happen if these were ignored. I hoped he would heed my advice.

I had borrowed some Petrea King meditation tapes from the Palliative Care library, and was finding them most helpful when I couldn't 'turn off' sufficiently to concentrate on my own meditating.

Petrea King is a natural therapies practitioner and qualified yoga and meditation teacher. In September 1983, she was diagnosed with an 'incurable' form of leukemia. Since her remarkable recovery, she has counselled many thousands of people and facilitated thousands of support groups for people with cancer and other life-threatening illnesses. Petrea lectures regularly on the role of natural therapies in cancer and palliative care.

I had the opportunity to attend a workshop she ran in conjunction with palliative care, and bought two of her books, *Quest for Life*, a handbook for people with life-threatening illness, and *Sometimes Hearts have to Break*, 25 inspirational journeys to healing and peace, which she signed for me. I also bought a range of her tapes, which I both used and lent to others. My buddy in Townsville particularly appreciated them.

Petrea King is a petite, quietly spoken woman, emanating peace and love. It's a privilege, pleasure and inspiration to be in her company.

I invited Bob for a weekend while he awaited his operation. He and I took a picnic to Mt Buffalo and had a gentle walk around the lake; Bob tired easily. I made him juice in lieu of his usual alcoholic beverage before dinner, which he surprised himself by enjoying, and we shared the preparation of a vegetable pasta sauce. He always refers to my diet as 'vegetarian muck', but none the less enjoys it.

He went into hospital for his bypass heart surgery two days later. I was so glad we had enjoyed that weekend together.

The appointment I had with my original oncologist was in rooms at the Royal Women's Hospital in Melbourne. Katrina offered to come with me. I knew it would mean a lot of organization on her part to get away for a full day (7.30am train to Melbourne, returning 8.30pm), leave Alex with someone, and arrange for Tom's after school care, but in the end I accepted.

I really needed and wanted a carer, and she sincerely wanted to be that special person for me.

My first instinct was to protect her from worry and inconvenience, but I decided not to do what Mum had always done to my sister and me, and that was to make her independence a barrier to the amount of love and care we could give her. Katrina was no longer a child I needed to protect, and she had a great network of friends to support her

I also decided to try and be easier on myself; I didn't need to be Wonder Women, just do my best.

Katrina and I made the most of our day in Melbourne. We saw a good movie, did some shopping, and had a gourmet lunch. We caught a taxi to the hospital, as we weren't sure how to get there on public transport.

What a totally different experience. I was once again thoroughly examined inside and out, the test results read, and the films viewed. The gyn/oncologist was quite confident the lesions on my liver were old cysts and not malignant. She said they never gave chemo on the strength of the blood test alone, and suggested that if it kept going up, I could try high-dose progesterone tablets, a hormone treatment that had proved successful in some cases. As long as I was feeling well, they wouldn't interfere. What a relief. Katrina asked some questions before we left, and I felt lighter and happier than I had in weeks.

The following weekend was spent in Wangaratta Ski Lodge, at Mt St. Bernard, from where the walking club did some fabulous walks around nearby Mt Hotham, enjoying the breath-taking views. I was determined to push cancer to the back of my mind and get back into life, and enjoy each day as it came.

The shadow of death

I travelled south late in February and spent some time with Mum doing a few things for her, then went on to Greg and Jane's where I stayed overnight and enjoyed special time with Samantha. The morning I was to travel home again, Anne, Ted's daughter rang me. She had been ringing my family looking for me with the news that Ted's health had suddenly deteriorated and he was in hospital. I thanked her for letting me know, and was on my way to the hospital before nine, battling the morning peak traffic.

When I arrived I found him in a private room semiconscious with labored breathing, a thready pulse and incontinent. His son and daughter-in-law were there, and Anne arrived soon after. She was very upset. The doctor couldn't explain Ted's sudden collapse, and had no idea what the next 24 hours would hold.

I sat with him holding his hand while Anne filled me in on the current state of affairs. I stayed for over an hour until others arrived, then kissed Ted goodbye, expecting it to be for the last time, and made a tearful exit.

On arriving home, I rang the hospital. Ted had died at 2.15pm.

I had planned to go away for the following week with the walking club, so I told Anne I would come to the funeral if it were on Friday, otherwise I would send flowers to go on his coffin. I did consider cancelling my trip, but two other members were relying on me for transport and the shared cost of accommodation. I decided Ted had controlled my life enough when alive, and I was not going to let it continue after his death.

I finally got the news that they planned to have Ted's

body cremated the following Wednesday, followed by a memorial service. They were going to release balloons with the names of the family members on them, which would include mine, Katrina's and Greg's.

During meditation the following morning, I was focusing on the pure, radiant love and light of God. I felt the presence of Ted in that radiance. I sensed that since he had been released from his diseased body and tortured mind, he was able to send pure love. What a surprise he must have got when he found death wasn't the total oblivion he had expected.

I felt moved to write to the girls and included the letter in a sympathy card. In part I said,

'Let all of us who loved and were loved by Ted remember the happy times and contemplate the reasons he came into our lives, and the lessons we learned from that for our own spiritual growth. Among other things, he brought me the experience and love of your family, for which I am very grateful. Weep for his physical, emotional and spiritual pain, but rejoice for the love he gave us on earth, and that he will always give us.'

I would like to have attended the service as a final farewell, and if I hadn't been able to actually say goodbye to him in the hospital, my decision would have been different.

When I returned from my walking holiday, it was to the great news that my sister Brenda had decided to move from suburban Blackburn to Healesville, to be closer to Mum. I was so relieved, as I felt I had deserted Mum and knew she sometimes felt alone and vulnerable. I was confident Brenda would enjoy living in picturesque Healesville, and Mum's quality of life would improve.

The roller-coaster ride continues

My CA-125 in March was 107, and my two-yearly bone scan showed my osteoporosis was worse, mainly in my spine. The termites arrived back in the laundry and were re-sprayed, Graham commenced another course of chemotherapy, and my friend Pauline's dear old Labrador departed this life; what a year so far!

April started on a much brighter note, with a bus trip to Melbourne with Lois to attend the International Flower and Garden Show, which we very much enjoyed.

Greg, Jane and Samantha came to stay over Easter, which that year coincided with Katrina's birthday. We had a family party, an Easter egg hunt, a big day cutting firewood with the usual barbecue in the paddock, and lots of tennis. How quiet the house seemed when they departed.

It was at this time I started drinking coffee again. I had been having headaches, something that had rarely bothered me in the last couple of years, so rather than take analgesics I tried a coffee. It worked, and it was delicious. The one-a-day habit I have now developed, I very much enjoy. To be able to meet a friend for coffee and actually have one, instead of herb tea, I find socially satisfying.

I attended a wonderful organ recital in the Wangaratta Cathedral with Doreen that month.

The sheep the farm manager had brought over from the main property to keep the grass down in the home paddock, started lambing. I could see them from the house without disturbing them, and the lambs were a delight to watch. Once they were a few days old, they would congregate in the late afternoon, and frolic and skip around together while their mums rested; I found myself laughing out loud at their antics.

On a more sober note, Mum had a skin cancer removed from her neck, which turned out to be a very painful procedure, and my OVCA buddy, J. in Townsville was deteriorating, with 'tumors popping up everywhere'. I wondered if that was how it would end up for me.

I was suffering more and more from fits of depression that year and was having trouble sleeping, and would become tearful over the least thing.

Rainbows

I spent a long and rejuvenating session with my guides one morning after hearing my buddy's news.

I let their love fill me, and sent love and healing to my distant friend; I then felt a lot more positive. I sent her an email and posted her a rainbow ribbon. I had learnt the concept of sending rainbows from Petrea King. The idea was to imagine the iridescent colors of the rainbow surrounding and permeating yourself (or everyone in the group if doing it in company). You take time to breathe in your favorite colors, then visualize the other end of the rainbow travelling across the sky to the person you have in mind. You then imagine the recipient bathed in the light and colors of the rainbow, giving them strength, peace, comfort and healing by the power of the rainbow. Petrea believes that just as you can have a vitamin deficiency, so you can have a rainbow deficiency, and I heartily agree (the same applies to hugs). Rainbows represent *being remembered with love*, and she believes that love has the power to heal all wounds. My buddy and I had a special time each day for sending each other rainbows.

I spent the remainder of the day in self-indulgence. I had the pedicure Katrina had given me a gift certificate for, treated myself to coffee and a French Vanilla slice at the bakery, and picked up the guinea pig hutch that was my birthday gift for Alex in a few days time. The day ended on a cheery note as I stayed with the boys for a couple of hours while Katrina attended a school meeting.

I bought the guinea pig itself the following day and settled it in the hutch with straw bedding, water and food. We had a lovely family party for Alex's second birthday, and he adored his new pet.

Early in May, I rang my OVCA buddy, K who was in Queensland undertaking a range of alternate therapies. Her CA-125 had jumped from 250 to 1,900 in a month. She was staying firm about her decision not to have further chemotherapy.

My CA-125 that month was up to 186, but I was feeling well physically, except for the headaches and some discomfort at times around my liver.

Feeling uncertain about the future, I decided to have some studio photos taken. I was usually the person behind the camera, so there were not a lot of photos of me around, and very few I approved of. I made an effort with my hair and carefully applied some makeup, and hoped for the best. The results were better than I had expected, so I chose my favorites and had them framed as gifts for family members.

A great break-through - as far as I was concerned - was the day Katrina and I had a conversation about my illness and I realized she had finally accepted that it was incurable, and she was even able to talk about my death. As far as I was concerned, her reluctance to talk about the inevitable, whenever it would be, had been a barrier in what was otherwise a very close relationship. With her acceptance I didn't feel quite so alone and afraid.

It was time to put some serious work into my holiday plans. Lord Howe Island with Pauline was off as she and her partner Fred decided on an overseas trip instead, so I revisited the travel agent for brochures and decided on a 20-day trip to Queensland in July. It included a bus trip from Sydney to Cairns, with all the usual tourist stops including Frazer and Hamilton Islands, culminating in a cruise from Cairns to Cooktown, Lizard Island and the outer reef. It would be the first time I had ever travelled alone, but I made friends easily and was confident I'd not be lonely. I paid the single supplement to have my own room rather than risk incompatible room-mates.

Katrina cooked me a lovely dinner for my birthday that year, and Alex made a great effort helping to blow out the candles.

Thank goodness I had Alex in my life with his bright, smiling face and infectious laugh. He loved to be left with me, and sometimes cried if Katrina called in and didn't leave him. He even stayed one night without Thomas.

Thomas and I continued our special times together at weekends and holidays. He was doing well at school and loved to do drawings and writing for me, and to demonstrate his reading prowess. The conversations during our early morning cuddles were important to us both. He was aware that his grandfather was very ill and possibly dying, and told me that I was getting older and my heart would stop one day too! I told him that Grandpa and I would always love him, even if we weren't here anymore. I feel you have to seize the moment for such conversations.

The Biggest Morning Tea was a resounding success that year; our muffins were becoming quite famous. I also enrolled to join a new Probus group in Wangaratta, along with Lois and Ivan and several friends from the walking group. I was finding the long walks too tiring, so this was a good way to stay in touch.

Greg and Jane had settled into their new home and it was time to tackle their garden, which was a hodge-podge of unrelated plants and broken edging. I offered my assistance and guidance, which was gladly accepted, and went and stayed with them for a few days, fitting in a visit to Mums and a look at Bren's new house at the same time.

Back home, it was the usual routine of keeping the fire going, housework, garden maintenance, minding the boys, and visiting clients. It should have been a full and satisfying life, but depression still plagued me. I was no longer meditating regularly, was less conscientious with my juices, and stopped taking Percy's powder. I don't know why specifically, it just seemed too much trouble.

A run of frustrating annoyances didn't help. Firstly the hot water service wasn't heating sufficiently (luke warm showers - yuk), and it took a variety of tradesmen to finally decide it needed a new time clock. Then my work-battered wheelbarrow needed replacing. Nothing as simple as buying a new one ready to use, it came in a thousand pieces definitely designed for more than one person to assemble.

Graham continued to deteriorate, and I urged his family to make use of the District Nursing Service, but they were not keen to do this. I was their unofficial Volunteer, but I was frustrated by the limited amount of help and advice I could give.

It was time for the annual interview and re-commitment as a Palliative Care Volunteer. As my present client was stable and coming off the Palliative Care list, I decided to retire from the service and concentrate on my own health issues. My CA-125 was up to 336, and my physician ordered a CT scan to see what was going on.

The scan was clear, and my other blood tests normal,

so he gave me his blessing to go on my holiday and was confident I'd stay well.

The day Katrina took me to the hospital for the scan, she took Alex to emergency to have a piece of popcorn removed from up his nose. It reminded me of an incident when Greg was about the same age and poked a 'Fruit Loop' up his nose. Why do children do that? My scan was over, and she was still waiting. They had to give Alex a sedative, then wait until that took effect, but they still couldn't retrieve the popcorn. He ended up needing a general anaesthetic the following day to have it removed.

That same day, we received the news that Graham now had a brain tumor. He was to try medication first to see if that helped, followed by radiotherapy.

Anne rang for a long chat and to say they were scattering Ted's ashes on the anniversary of his birthday. I would be in Queensland at that time, so would miss out once more. I asked if I could have a small quantity of his ashes for my own ceremony.

My buddy, K. was home from Queensland, and I caught up with her at home via the phone. She had to talk to me with an oxygen mask on. The cancer was eating away her lungs, and she had severe ascites (fluid in the abdominal cavity). I arranged to visit the following Wednesday, not even sure she'd last that long. I was very upset, not just for her and her son, who I had got to know, but also in relation to my own death and myself. She had spent thousands of dollars on her relocation and treatment, and had pursued a huge range of alternative treatments, all to no avail. My buddy, J. in Townsville was also fighting a losing battle despite all the medical treatment; why did I think I'd be the exception to the rule and beat this insidious disease, as it would obviously win in the end.

I rang on the Tuesday evening before my planned visit

to K. Her mother answered the phone and told me K. was in hospital with a partial bowel obstruction, and asked me not to visit – family only. K died the following day, just 18 months after diagnosis. The funeral was to be held in Sydney, so all I could do was send a card expressing my condolence, and inviting her son to keep in touch if he needed to talk.

Thomas came down with chicken pox.

Holiday magic

The day came at last for departing on my holiday. Tom was still home from school convalescing, and Alex was off colour. Katrina drove me to Albury airport for my flight to Sydney to join the tour.

The flight was nearly half an hour late due to fog in Melbourne, but it was no trouble keeping the boys occupied watching the planes coming and going. When it was finally time to board, Tom hung around my neck saying, "I'll miss you too much". We were both crying. Luckily, I had a window seat to divert my attention to the snow-capped Alps that came into view shortly after take off, which settled me into holiday mode.

I successfully collected my luggage on landing, and located the airport bus that dropped me at the hotel. My room overlooked Darling Harbor, very nice. I spent the afternoon exploring The Rocks with a friend living in Sydney, and was up before dawn the next day to join the tour.

We soon drove out of the rain and into fine weather, which would stay with us for the rest of the trip North.

Coff's Harbour and Byron Bay were picture perfect, and Frazer and Hamilton Islands were a great contrast, both beautiful in their own way. I was totally enchanted with the Reef, and viewed it in three different locations.

While passing through Townsville, I had arranged to

meet my buddy J. and her husband. He picked me up from the hotel late in the afternoon, and took me to the hospital to visit her. We had been sending hugs to each other via email for months, so it was great to at last share the real thing. J. was bald, pale, thin and pot-bellied, but bright as a button. We chatted for well over an hour, then she wanted her husband to take me to see their home, a lovely 1950s 'Queenslander' he was renovating, high on a hill overlooking the town. What a lovely, caring man he was. We talked about his expectations over the coming weeks, and I urged him to keep in touch with me when J. was beyond communicating with me herself.

He drove me back to the hotel, where I joined my fellow travellers for dinner. I was glad to be offered a nice glass of wine to drown my sorrows.

The three-day cruise from Cairns to Cooktown, Lizard Island and the outer reef was wonderful, and would have been even better if I could have shared it with someone special. I flew from Cairns to Sydney; then changed planes to Albury.

My connecting flight was delayed due to bad weather, so I was half an hour late arriving. Two very excited little boys greeted me, and Tom insisted on carrying my heavy backpack to the car. I gave them their gifts, and they were both asleep when Rob dropped me home. Katrina, who was working that evening, had got the fire going and put food in the fridge for me, which I very much appreciated. I slept like a baby in my own comfy bed.

It had been a most wonderful luxurious holiday, visiting all the places I had longed to see. The food was consistently delicious, the accommodation very comfortable, and the company great. There was a very big hole in my bank account, but it was worth every cent.

It was back to reality with a frosty morning the next day. I picked Meg up from the cattery, and she was very pleased to be home; I even think the chooks were happy to see me.

When I called in to see Katrina and have a hug and give her and Rob their gifts, Alex demonstrated the progress he had made with his speech and said 'Mummy' instead of just 'Mum', and, 'Love you Ma Ma', making it a perfect home-coming.

Graham had continued to deteriorate despite the radiotherapy, but was battling on, determined to see that year's calves born and recorded as part of Breedplan. He had founded his Wyuna Poll Hereford Stud in Byawatha in 1955, and in 1980, was the Chairman of the newly founded Northeast Poll Hereford Breeders Group. Some of his cattle were listed in the top 10% in Australia. He also gave his time generously to Rotary over many years, and was recently awarded a life membership.

He had always supported his four children with their numerous school and sporting activities, and was a valued member of the local Uniting Church. He was truly one of nature's gentlemen, and it tore at my heart to see him so low.

The 4th of August was Brenda's moving day; it was also the anniversary of Dad's birthday. During the stressful time of house hunting, she had been in touch with Dad, and he had assured her that everything would work out okay. I wondered if Mum had seen the significance of Brenda moving closer to her on that particular day, as a message from Dad.

Graham's health and strength deteriorated rapidly during August. He had chosen to die at home, and the family cared for him as best they could with the support of the District Nursing Service and Palliative Care. I supported and comforted his loving sister Marj, and offered my advice and services to the rest of the family if needed.

I had the privilege of sitting with Graham as he lapsed into unconsciousness. His devoted old dog was very distressed, so I ended up with one hand on her, and one on Graham, giving them Reiki, which brought peace to them both. Graham remained in a coma for the next 48 hours, before dying peacefully at home with his dog by his side.

Sadly, Rob interpreted my assistance as interference, and it has created a barrier between us ever since. I had done nothing without first seeking permission from both Graham and Lesley, so my conscience was clear, but his attitude towards me was still very distressing.

I escaped to Greg and Jane's for a couple of days before the funeral, and found that Sam had grown and changed a lot since I'd last seen her in May. The best and most wonderful news was that they were expecting another baby the following March.

Graham's funeral was very well attended, proof of the high esteem with which he was held in the community. As soon as Alex saw me, he insisted on sitting with me during the service. Thomas was being very grown up and was sitting with the rest of the family, complete with collar and tie. He had coped very maturely through the previous few days, insisting on seeing Grandpa's dead body, and on going to the Crematorium, but over the following months would often be found sitting on the couch 'feeling sad', or crying because he missed Grandpa.

During the night a couple of days after Graham's death, Katrina woke to see a man standing at the end of their bed. Terrified, she screamed and he disappeared. Awake enough by then to assess the situation, she realised it was probably Graham visiting Rob, and still sobbing, she kept saying "Sorry Graham" while Rob, awakened by the noise, comforted her. She regretted so much frightening Graham's spirit away at that time, but her reaction was a very natural one. At least she is now prepared if I choose to visit her in spirit, and hopefully she will not be so surprised and frightened.

Time for action

By September, my CA-125 was up to 604. I rang for an appointment with my physician for later in the month, with the aim of finding out where the cancer was active, as not knowing was driving me crazy. I didn't particularly want treatment, but needed to have some idea what symptoms I could expect. As the appointment wasn't for three weeks, I rang my gyn/oncologist in Melbourne and had a satisfying talk about my condition.

She suggested I try the high dose progesterone tablets (an hormonal form of chemotherapy), as she had patients with the same type of tumor who had experienced good results. I told her that quality, not quantity of life was my priority, and she said she understood. I was to have another CA-125 immediately prior to starting the progesterone, for which she would post me a prescription.

September 12th. When I turned on the radio for the early news, it was to hear of the terrorist attack in New York. I was appalled, and concerned for my OVCA buddy residing in that city. I emailed her and anxiously awaited a reply; she was safe, but badly shaken emotionally.

My appetite had dwindled and I could only eat small meals without feeling nauseated, and I wasn't sure if it was the effect of the cancer or just my anxiety and depression about it. I was also having some trouble with constipation and experiencing odd bouts of abdominal pain. It was time for another session with Trisha to get myself back on track.

I had been reading a book called *The Journey*, by Brandon Bays. In 1992, Brandon was diagnosed with a football-sized tumor and found herself catapulted into a remarkable, soul-searching and ultimately freeing healing journey. Six and a half weeks later she was pronounced perfectly well, without the aid of drugs or surgery. Brandon's book outlines her personal story, then, through a series of workshops, guides the reader to the root cause of any longstanding difficulty. She then gives them the tools to finally and completely resolve it.

Trisha had read the book, and I discussed it with her and asked if she'd help lead me on a journey within my own body. She agreed, and it was very revealing. During my journey I dredged up a lot of old feelings, and worked on my self worth.

It was emotionally draining, but most therapeutic. Trisha made up some Bach flower essence drops for me to take home to help stabilise me emotionally.

The 'script for the Provera (progesterone) came, and I commenced taking the tablets in the middle of September. Greg had looked up all the information he could find about them on the web and emailed it to me, which I found most helpful. I just hoped I was doing the right thing taking this drug, considering the possible side effects.

Four days after commencing Provera, I started getting headaches from an intense feeling of pressure in my head. These headaches became a regular part of my life, night and day, and turned out to be from high blood pressure – up to 175 as a side effect of the drug. My normal blood pressure was around 125. A couple of weeks later I developed a chronic cough that kept me awake night after night, and disrupted any conversation I tried to conduct.

I was back on a roundabout of drugs to combat the affect of other drugs, and I was not happy about it.

Meanwhile, my buddy in Townsville was deteriorating and wasn't able to speak to me when I rang, so I kept up the emails and continued to send her love and healing when I meditated.

On the 19th of September her husband rang to say J's kidneys had failed and she was coming home to die. By the 23rd she was semi-comatosed, and she died peacefully at home surrounded by family and friends two days later. I wept for the loss of a special friend; I'm sure we'll meet again.

An unexpected surprise was a weekend visit by Greg, Jane and Samantha, with Jane's parents Eric and Rosemary joining us for some of the time. The cousins were happily reunited, and the adults played lots of tennis. Samantha's favorite job was collecting the eggs, and she checked the nests every half-hour or so.

As usual, I was feeling rather flat when the house was empty again and had the urge to update my will and print out some of my writing to leave for Katrina and Greg. I also went through my CD collection and wrote down the titles of some of my favorite music and why it was special to me. This gave me solace.

I had been working conscientiously in my garden preparing the vegetable patch for summer planting, and mulching the beds before the anticipated heat, always good therapy for depression, but my sciatica started troubling me again, so it was back to the chiropractor for more regular treatments. I was constantly nauseated and didn't know if it was from the cancer or the Provera, but I battled on, enjoying the boys' company and unconditional love whenever I got the chance.

America launched war against the Taliban in Afghanistan

in early October, and I avoided watching the news telecasts, I was so appalled.

October was also the month for the annual school sports day, Tom's first such event. He performed with more enthusiasm than skill, as most of the prep children did, and had a wonderful day. Alex participated in the toddler race and was swept along in the crowd of encouraging older siblings. A very happy day.

Later that month, an Open Garden Day to aid the local school was held, and I was one of the participants. Ivan and Lois had helped me hang some of their youngest daughter's beautiful quilts in my enclosed back verandah on the Friday, to add to the display created by my garden in its full spring glory.

A steady stream of visitors over three hours seemed to appreciate both the garden and the quilts, and I had some very interesting botanical discussions, and learnt some history about the property and the family that had established it.

I was scheduled for a CT scan the next day. It was routine, and Katrina had me home again by lunchtime, then Bob arrived for an overnight stay on his long trip to Western Australia for a family reunion, coinciding with Christmas. He was on the road to his big adventure in good time the next morning, stocked with preserves and a fruitcake I had made for him.

Later that day, I picked up the films from the scan and went to see my GP for the results. There was nothing showing, and my CA-125 was 625. It had been 580 when I started the Provera, so at least it had stabilized. Perhaps it would be worth the side effects, though the high blood pressure readings were a real concern.

I had heard many good reports about a Chinese Herbalist practising in Albury, 40kms away, so I decided to consult him to see if he could help control the side affects and symptoms I was experiencing. I had written a comprehensive medical history and diet and medication sheet to take with me, which he appreciated. Working with him was a nurse who was studying herbal medicine and was doing practical placement there. The herbalist's accent was very heavy, so I was glad of her interpretations. I was given a half-hour acupuncture treatment, something I hadn't experienced before, and came away with a weeks supply of herbs to take. I brewed up a pot of the herbs when I got home and found them revolting, but was determined to persevere in the hope it was an acquired taste. It wasn't, but I kept brewing them twice a day until I saw him again the following week.

He was both amazed and delighted at my progress. My blood pressure and cough were still a problem, but my intestines had cleared and the pain I had been experiencing, disappeared. Following another acupuncture treatment, I went home with a further two weeks supply of herbs. I consumed these as prescribed, but as they were so utterly horrible to take, and I felt they had done all they could, I did not return for more.

The Melbourne Cup holiday weekend was filled with the usual happy family experiences of shared meals and fun together, as Greg and Jane had come to stay. They gave Thomas a junior tennis racket for his birthday, and Greg spent several patient hours giving him lessons. Once more, Thomas had more enthusiasm than skill, but was already making progress after a couple of days. I captured the highlights of the long weekend on video, which lightened my mood when I replayed them when once again alone in my big empty house.

Thomas's sixth birthday party was a riotous affair

as all his schoolmates raced around the garden, with Katrina and I trying to organise games and food. I for one was relieved when their parents picked up the guests a couple of hours later. The family arrived for a more sedate evening celebration, and two very tired little boys were tucked into bed that night.

My CA-125 result a few days later was 797; so much for the Provera working. I consulted my physician the following week and he insisted it was time to see an oncologist again. The thought of traipsing into Melbourne was more than I could face, so he referred me to an oncologist in Wodonga, an easy drive away.

I was pretty upset and had a cry when I got home. When Katrina called around later, I shared the day's events and we clung to each other in a supportive embrace, and she offered to accompany me to Wodonga. She was a bit depressed herself following the disappointing news that the long-awaited, much planned, and desperately needed house extension and renovation had been postponed indefinitely, right on the brink of its inception.

The next day I had the diversion of a 4WD trip with some Probus members, another first time experience. We had lunch in the beautiful Howqua Valley, and it was a most exciting and enjoyable day in great company.

Greg rang me that evening and told me the firm he worked for were shedding thousands of employees, and to retain the job he had meant competing with two mates he had worked closely with for many years. It was a worrying prospect that he might lose his job just as the new baby was due. Something else to add to my list of worries in this horrible year.

Then my car broke down and was only running on three cylinders. The mechanic said it could be for various reasons, some of them major and very expensive to repair, but he wouldn't know until he took a look. It turned out to be something relatively minor and not too expensive, much to my relief.

December brought with it the anticipation of Christmas celebrations with family and friends. The pudding had been made weeks before and was maturing in a cool, dark cupboard. Gifts were hidden in the top of the wardrobe, and cards and wrapping purchased. Jam was bottled and decoratively labelled along with shortbread, mince tarts, truffles and Christmas cake.

My annual weekend at Anglesea with Margot and Joan was in doubt as Margot's Mum was unwell, but in the end we took her along with us and we all enjoyed a restful, chatty weekend in the fresh sea air.

On the 10th of December, Katrina and I travelled to Wodonga for my appointment with the oncologist. She seemed very nice, a straight talker, but kind. She made it clear there was no cure for ovarian cancer, and treatment only put off the inevitable. I glanced over at Katrina to see how she was coping with this no-frills approach; she seemed calm. Chemotherapy was my only option if I chose treatment, and the oncologist suggested I have the same drugs as last time as they had been so effective.

She didn't expect to get my CA-125 below 200 this time, and wanted me to start the chemotherapy course that week. I said I'd prefer to leave it until after Christmas, and she agreed. The 3rd of January was decided on. This time the dosage was based on a blood test to ascertain kidney function, and my present weight. This worked out to be a lower dose than I had previously had, so I optimistically hoped it would mean less severe side effects. I left with a prescription for antibiotics to hopefully clear up my persistent cough, and one each for the strongest anti nausea drug, and some sleeping tablets. I was to cease taking Provera a week before commencing the new chemotherapy regime.

I rang the family with the latest news and to discuss Christmas arrangements. As Rob would be too busy harvesting to come down to join in the celebrations, Katrina and I had planned travelling together in her car with the boys. While trying to work out transport arrangements for our family gathering, my sister Brenda and I had an unfortunate misunderstanding which got blown out of proportion through lack of communication, and almost caused Mum to decide not to join us for dinner. I soothed the troubled waters as best I could, but the atmosphere was tense on the day.

I pushed the entire emotional trauma aside and tried not to think about the impending chemo, and concentrated on the good things.

Katrina purchased a fresh pine tree, and the boys had great fun decorating it. I put out my decorations, including the musical ones that played carols, and the house rang with Christmas joy whenever Katrina and the boys came over. This was quite regularly, as Katrina's oven was still awaiting parts to repair it with.

The Christmas recital at the Wangaratta Cathedral was delightful, and the walking club social gathering, held at Ivan and Lois's was fun, but the school concert was the highlight.

The items had been shrouded in a veil of secrecy that Thomas wouldn't reveal, but he was very nervous and teary when it was time to go to the hall. He didn't participate much at first, but when *Bob the Builder* was sung he really got into the swing of it and was the star performer. I think seeing me with the video camera helped. The evening culminated with the arrival of Santa, and all the children, including younger siblings such as Alex, received a gift. That was when Alex realised that Santa meant gifts, and he was really caught up in the excitement.

Katrina picked Tom up after his final day at school for the year, and we travelled down to Melbourne to celebrate Christmas. We had afternoon tea with Mum, and then Katrina and the boys went on to visit other friends.

The following morning, Mum and I chatted over breakfast as we usually did when I visited, and she insisted I tell her all that the oncologist had said. I put it as honestly and gently as I could, knowing that was what she wanted. We hugged before she went off to get ready for our Christmas luncheon. Katrina picked us up late morning, and Samantha was most excited to see the boys, and more cousins as the extended family soon joined them.

It was a buffet meal, and the different family groups kept themselves apart from each other. I drifted from group to group but felt I might just as well have been in spirit looking on. Gift opening was a riot of torn paper and over excitement, nobody really knowing what had come from whom.

At dusk, when all the other guests had departed and the three children bathed, I went for a walk along the nearby streets with my children and grandchildren, to view the houses festooned with lights and other Christmas decorations. Thomas was enchanted and wanted to spend the rest of Christmas there.

Back home, I spent Christmas Eve visiting friends with small gifts from my kitchen, culminating at Pauline's for a relaxing drink.

Christmas day was the coldest in Victoria since 1924. I awoke at five and wondered if the boys were awake, and learnt later that Thomas had been up before six, and Alex an hour later.

It was a long, lonely day for me. I was invited to the cottage for the evening meal, so I spent Christmas lunch alone for the first time in my life, and was miserable. The cold, wet weather didn't help. I prepared myself a prawn and mango salad and had a glass of wine and some pudding I had brought back from Greg and Jane's, and filled the day watching old movies on TV.

Katrina finally rang after six to say it was convenient to come around, so I loaded the car with gifts and food. The boys were still having their afternoon sleep, and Rob was out on the farm somewhere when I arrived. The boys finally awoke and I gave them their gifts, and we ate dinner at nine. Rob was barely civil to me and ignored the gifts I gave him. Katrina was exhausted, so I washed up for her and went home at 10.30, feeling less than joyous. I wrote in my journal, ' On reflection, this Christmas was mostly about presents and food, with very little family fellowship. People gathered and gestures were made, but seemed to lack warmth and depth. I don't want another Christmas like this. If I can't gather around a table as a family to talk and laugh, and honestly be glad to be together, forget it'.

On Boxing Day, the chooks got into the garden and scratched off all the mulch, making a terrible mess. I chased them out, screaming and yelling; thank goodness I don't have close neighbors. I found some wire netting and patched the hole they had come through, then spent a quiet evening in the depths of misery.

I was hurt and angry about Rob's behavior, and apprehensive about the rapidly approaching chemotherapy treatment. I wished I hadn't committed to it, as I felt I wanted to die before next Christmas.

A day in the garden had its usual calming effect the next day, and I took myself to the movies to divert my mind when I went shopping the following day. I filled the remaining days of the old year with major household and garden chores that I didn't anticipate being able to do while on chemo.

I invited Katrina around for a chat one evening, just the two of us. As we sipped a Bailey's, I asked her if she knew the reason for Rob's attitude towards me, and if it was causing conflict in their relationship. She explained that as far as she knew he was still holding a grudge from when his father was dying, but it was not interfering with the relationship between her and me. I found this hard to believe. I tried to explain how depressed I was feeling and why, and she suggested I needed professional help; perhaps she was right. I felt better for our chat, even if she didn't. What a mess.

Bob had been ringing intermittently from Western Australia where he had enjoyed a great time with his family, and I was anticipating a visit before the New Year, on his way home. He didn't turn up. Perhaps unreasonably, I felt let down. I had told him that I was starting chemotherapy in early January and was feeling apprehensive and depressed and in need of a friend and a supportive shoulder to cry on. I suppose I was reaping what I had sown when I insisted on a less intimate relationship a couple of years earlier.

The last day of the old year was spent with Katrina and the boys on our annual excursion to the Berry Farm in Stanley. Thomas ate so many berries he was sick, and both their faces were stained purple. We enjoyed a delicious lunch at the Beechworth Bakery before coming home.

Ivan and Lois picked me up at 8pm to spend the evening at the local Italian Club to see the New Year in. It was a friendly evening of dancing and talking, with a delicious supper and champagne at midnight.

Four significant people in my life had died that year, and I had lived with my own cancer time bomb ticking, and the future looked bleak.

My New Year's resolution was to find a reason for living that was worth fighting for.

Chapter 6

The Final countdown - Quality vs. quantity

More Chemotherapy

Two days until the re-commencement of chemotherapy. Packing up Christmas decorations and getting the washing up to date kept me occupied, and Thomas jumped at the invitation to stay the night. We had decided not to tell him what was happening to me yet; he was still grieving for his grandfather. Katrina would just keep the boys away from me while I was recovering from chemo and was looking and feeling ghastly.

Thomas and I enjoyed our time together playing cards and having stories before bed, then our early morning cuddle and pancakes for breakfast.

Dropping him home mid morning, I went on to take Megan to the vets for her annual booster injection, then to stock up on fresh fruit and high-dose anti oxidant tablets. I also went to pathology for a blood test. The evening was spent thoroughly watering the garden.

Thursday 3rd January. Chemo day dawned. I had slept better than expected, and enjoyed a sustaining breakfast before packing a book, my Walkman and some fruit juice to take with me. Katrina delivered me to the oncology unit and waited at home for a phone call several hours later to pick me up.

It took a couple of attempts to find a vein before I was

given the usual pre-chemo drugs, including the strongest anti-nausea drug. During the last saline flush following the second bag of chemo, my vein started aching and the nurse applied a soothing warm compress.

Once home, I was happy to spend the remainder of the day relaxing in my recliner, diverted by a video. Bob rang during the evening, and he sounded surprised to hear I had started chemo that day. By taking the most direct route from the West, he had arrived home on the 30th of December, in time to spend the New Year with his friends at Venus Bay. I guessed I now knew where I stood in his priority of friends. They certainly would have been more fun to be with.

After taking the prescribed anti-nausea tablets and suppositories, I went to bed with a bowl by my side 'just in case'.

My vein continued to ache and reflux prevented me lying comfortably, and sleep evaded me, despite sleeping tablets. The vomiting started about 6am, and in a way it was a relief, as it eased the pressure and bloating I was feeling. Katrina came around while I had a shower, and made the bed for me. I snacked on fruit and drank as much as I could during the day, trying to flush out the chemo and keep hydrated, but I was feeling like a zombie, and all my joints ached. I rubbed Tiger Balm into them and took paracetamol and hoped I'd sleep.

By Saturday, the nausea was no longer a problem, but I had developed abdominal pain, which was most uncomfortable and kept me awake. I was only eating small amounts of nourishing food to keep my strength up, but the pain got progressively worse. I took a laxative in case it was merely constipation.

I awoke shortly after midnight Sunday morning in a sweat, my heart racing; loneliness and fear threatened to overtake me. I pulled myself together, and after taking my temperature and finding it elevated, took two paracetamol and some drops of Rescue Remedy, a Bach flower blend that calms the nerves, and did some Reiki on myself.

I dozed fitfully until 4am, when my temperature was still elevated and the pain persisted. How much worse everything feels at night.

The laxative worked well when I arose at six, then I went back to bed for a couple of hours. My abdomen was still bloated and tender, which was a worry. I felt so vulnerable all alone in my big house.

I decided to take up my physician's offer to ring him anytime, so feeling in need of his advice, I rang his mobile number. He was on holiday at the seaside, and he advised me to go to the hospital as my temperature was elevated. Katrina wasn't home, so I left a message and called an ambulance.

After spending three uncomfortable hours in emergency having blood and urine tests and an X-ray, the tests were inconclusive, and I was told my symptoms were just a reaction to the chemo and I'd have to tolerate them until they wore off!

Katrina brought me home and stayed until I had some fruit, jelly and custard and was feeling a little better. I pottered about watering plants and returning phone calls; Mum was very worried about me. I took paracetamol again before retiring for the night.

Monday morning, I awoke at two with my belly on fire and an elevated temperature. Fear gripped me and I called for Dad and felt his loving presence, which calmed me down a little. Analgesics and a sleeping pill got me through the remainder of the night.

On ringing my oncologist later in the morning, I found that she too was away on holiday. Her partner in the practice rang me back later and said the abdominal pain had nothing to do with the chemo, and to see my GP to be examined.

Pauline drove me to the surgery, and as my usual doctor was also on holiday, I saw a locum. The examination was inconclusive, so she spoke to the oncologist who suggested an ultrasound, which was booked for the following day.

I had a better night Tuesday with the aid of analgesics, and I managed a few light chores during the day. I found a dead snake by the front gate and started to worry that Meg had killed it and been bitten in the process. I hadn't seen her all morning, and my imagination took flight, which ended in tears.

During the ultrasound that afternoon, the technician let it slip that there were polyps in my gall bladder, which sounded ominous, so I was anxious to discuss it with a doctor. At least I now knew the source of the pain.

Megan greeted me on my return and I gathered her into my arms and hugged her. She had been so comforting and affectionate over the last few days, I just couldn't bear the thought of losing her, particularly now.

On Wednesday night, analgesics assisted my sleep once more, until I awoke at 4.30am with a searing pain at the base of my skull, radiating into my head, the like of which I'd never experienced before. The strongest analgesics brought absolutely no relief, and the stabbing pain in my head nearly drove me crazy. My scalp was so tender I couldn't touch it, and lying down made it worse, so I just sat in bed in the dark rocking and crying for two hours. Exhausted, I took two sleeping pills and dozed through the pain for a while. A coffee at eight finally eased it.

After trying unsuccessfully to ring my chiropractor, thinking it was a problem with my neck, I finally rang Katrina and pleaded for help.

She had a friend who was a practising chiropractor in Benalla, half an hours drive away, and she arranged for me to see her as soon as we could get there.

I had a shower while I waited for Katrina to pick me up, feeling totally spaced out after all the pain and drugs. Coby, the chiropractor, made some adjustments and did a lot of networking (energy work), and I felt more relaxed and was pain-free when we left half an hour later. I spent the remainder of the day quietly at home. Lois called around with flowers, which cheered me up somewhat. Retiring to bed that night, I prayed the head pain would not return.

At 1am, I awoke in a sweat with the pain back in my head. Trying to stay calm, I took two Panadeine, lit my oil burner, made a cup of relaxing herb tea and sat in my recliner for an hour until the pain started to ease. Returning to bed, I dozed until 6.30, then had a coffee to clear my head.

I managed a little housework during the day, and picked roses for the house, and for Pauline. Her three dogs had 'gone bush' and she was worried sick about them. Fred, despite an infected leg, was out for hours on end searching for them. Coby was visiting Katrina that afternoon, so I made her a sweet-smelling posy of herbs, and took it to her after seeing Pauline.

The doctor rang with the results of the ultrasound; no metastasis on the liver or stones in the gall bladder, just cholesterol polyps (benign). My CA-125 reading immediately before commencing chemotherapy had been 1220.

When I rang Greg that evening with a current health report, he was sounding very frazzled. They were trying to upgrade Samantha into a bed from her cot, and she wouldn't settle.

The headache started that night before I could escape into sleep, and persisted for eight hours. I thought I'd go crazy. If I'd been near a cliff I'd have jumped off it!

On seeing my usual chiropractor the following afternoon, he explained that the pain I was experiencing was cluster headaches, a form of migraine, which was a cerebral disturbance brought on by stress, and usually lasted about a week. He suggested a different type of analgesic, Nurophen, which I purchased before going home. He also did some work on my neck and head that he hoped would help.

A pain-free night at last. I felt like a new woman, and did two loads of washing and baked berry muffins, which the boys and Katrina enjoyed when they visited. It was so lovely to see the boys again.

Over the following days, I picked up strength, and only had mild headaches, which I could control. It was so great to be living more normally again. This chemo had better work - and work well - I thought.

On seeing my physician two weeks after commencing chemotherapy, I told him my tale of woe and he said I should have got an ambulance to hospital every time I had pain! He arranged for the palliative care nurses to call in and see me following my next dose of chemotherapy, and said he would add an anti-anxiety drug to my list of medications. The next session was due the Thursday before the Australia Day long weekend. I discussed the possibility of postponing it until the Tuesday after, so that if I needed help it would be available, and he agreed it was a good idea. I went through the wig catalogue that afternoon and chose one I liked, and sent off a sample of my hair for color matching. If I lost my hair this time, it would just be a matter of making a phone call and the wig would arrive promptly by express mail. I hoped I wouldn't have to make that call.

By the **19th** I was starting to feel more like my old self and was eating and sleeping better, and not needing an afternoon nap. I went to the local water hole and watched the boys swim, and attended the monthly Probus club meeting.

While feeding the chooks one evening, I suddenly saw a five-foot brown snake stretched out in the corner of the pen. I beat a hasty retreat and shut the door, and rang Katrina to see if Rob was around to dispose of it for me. He was out in the paddock, but she said she'd ring him and get back to me. Meanwhile, I donned heavy boots and armed myself with the long handled spade. Rob arrived promptly, but there was no sign of the snake in the pen where I had seen it. We found it in an adjacent pen with its head down a hole. Rob shot it in the back, then I held it down with a shovel while he dug its head out and gave it a final whack to make sure it was dead. Thomas was a very interested witness to this drama and couldn't wait to pick up the corpse, quite unafraid. Snakes have always been part of his life. We draped the body over a fence, and after thanking Rob, I went inside and had a Baileys to calm me down.

The law in Australia protects snakes, and I'm not afraid of snakes in the bush, but I'm not fond of meeting them in a confined space. Brown snakes are the second most toxic in the world despite having very short fangs, so I considered protecting myself, Megan, the chooks and my visitors from future encounters, worth breaking the law for.

The chooks were loath to go into their pen that night.

True to his word, the physician had notified the palliative care service of my need.

The co-ordinater, a nurse I knew from when I was a volunteer, came to visit, and we chatted for an hour and a half. It was so good to be able to talk freely about my depression and fears to someone who understood.

I had an appointment later in January to see the oncologist. Lesley looked after the boys so Katrina and I had one of our rare days alone together. We planned combining the appointment with some shopping and lunch. The oncologist said she had no idea why I had experienced so much abdominal pain as it was not a known side effect, and said that if it happened again she would discontinue the treatment. My blood cells had all recovered and were back to normal, and my CA-125 was already down to 293 after the first dose. She agreed to leave the next dose until after the long weekend, though she was not happy about the delay, but, as the treatment was 'only palliative', it wouldn't matter! I didn't appreciate her negative attitude.

Katrina and I did our shopping and I bought a gift for my new grandchild, the main reason I was prepared to undergo chemotherapy.

Even though I had a few extra days grace, I started getting depressed at the thought of the next chemo session and the pain that might follow, especially the headaches. A most wonderful surprise saved the day. Greg rang to see if it was convenient for them to come up and stay the weekend; I suspected Katrina had something to do with it. I jumped at the offer. I could now throw myself into cooking in preparation for their arrival.

On Friday, I had a lovely time with the boys while Katrina did her mowing. We made fishing lines with sticks and string and dug up worms to tie on the ends. Down by the creek, we feasted on blackberries while we 'fished'.

The boys stripped off and had a splash, and made dams and all those other lovely things children do with water. Oh to be a child again!

The weekend was wonderful. Tennis was confined to the cool of the evenings, and swimming in the mine was very popular.

After my visitors departed, I filled the remaining day before the dreaded chemotherapy by taking the boys to the movies to see *Monsters Inc.* It was Alex's first trip to the movies, and he loved it, as he munched his way through a tub of popcorn. Housework and gardening occupied the rest of the day.

I was feeling calmer than expected when I awoke on the day of my second dose of chemo. A chatty phone call from my old friend Margot, filled the time well until Katrina picked me up for my 10am date with the oncology nurse. The needle went in first try this time, and I was given extra saline on completion of the chemotherapy, leaving me well hydrated. The nurses had been giving extra IV fluid to the chemo patients, and were finding they were doing and feeling a lot better for it. I was happy to participate in the experiment. The physician had forgotten to order the extra drugs for anxiety.

My vein became inflamed again, but the application of warm packs and emu oil eased it. The prescribed regime of anti-nausea drugs failed to keep the reflux, nausea and vomiting at bay, so I felt pretty terrible the next day. Katrina came around while I showered, and the district nurse called in at lunchtime. There was nothing she could do, but she invited me to ring if I had any problems. I snoozed, and ate and drank small amounts during the day, and the nausea still plagued me.

The abdominal pain didn't return this time, but the headaches were occurring both day and night. Knowing the warning signs, I found that if I took Nurophen right at the start, I could cut down the duration of the pain to one or two hours, which was a vast improvement on the previous eight.

Four days later I was still nauseated, headachy and depressed, and decided I wanted to quit chemo. I made an appointment with my physician to tell him. The next time I spoke to Mum, I told her I was considering discontinuing chemotherapy, and she was very understanding, but Katrina was less enthusiastic when informed.

Lois called in and caught me feeling sorry for myself, and I got a bit teary when she hugged me. She offered to take me to visit Mum one day if I wanted to; what wonderful friends I have.

The decision to quit gave me a new lease on life and I did some baking for Katrina, who was still without the use of her oven. She came around later with fresh corn from her garden and to have a shower, as their bath was full of yabbies waiting to be prepared and eaten! She was quite upset about my decision to discontinue chemo, and I hoped we'd get a chance to sit down quietly in the near future to discuss it.

Pauline called in and we talked about our mutual need to have a purposeful and positive project in our lives. We understood each other so well, both being prone to depression and needing more than a daily routine to give purpose to living. We discussed many possibilities including joining a political party such as the Greens. Nothing felt really right. The district nurse rang to see how I was feeling, and I went to sleep to the welcome sound of rain on the roof. It was milder than usual that summer, but still hot and dry most of the time.

One of the oncology nurses rang the next day, and we discussed my negative attitude to chemotherapy. She knew Katrina through the school as they both had children attending there, and she offered to visit Katrina and give her the opportunity to express how she was feeling; I was very grateful.

I spent a lot of time that day assessing the priorities in my life, and wrote in my journal that night; 'The most important aspects of my life include love; to love and be loved by someone special, I no longer had that; to be an integral part of my extended family; I didn't have that anymore. Mum has Brenda, and Brenda and I hardly ever talk, and my brother doesn't want to know us. Greg has his own life in Melbourne, and I am not included in Katrina's family events anymore because of Rob's feelings towards me. I must make my own life and enjoyment with friends, but I need to be feeling well to do that, so I am willing to take the gamble and enjoy the here and now and do the walks and outings already planned, and take the future as it comes. I'll run out of money soon anyway then feel miserable, so nobody is going to talk me into chemo again. I'll be very sad if Katrina can't see my point of view, and only her own, but it's up to her.'

Turning Point

The following day proved to be a full and eventful one. I met friends from the walking club in Wangaratta, and we had coffee together and planned what food we'd take with us to Mt St Bernard in two weekend's time. I then went to Trisha's for a massage. On her table was a program for the year's courses at the local TAFE College. Both she and her husband were doing single subjects in the writing course.

'What a good idea', I thought, and following my massage, I returned to Wangaratta and inquired about enrolments. I made an appointment to speak to a tutor later that day, and returned home for lunch, my mind buzzing.

My GP rang to see what had been happening with my treatment, and she said she would support me with whatever I decided to do. I called in to see Katrina on my way back to Wangaratta. Alex was asleep so we were able to have a good talk. The oncology nurse had visited for coffee and a chat, and it had obviously been most beneficial.

As we talked, I realised I had changed my attitude and accepted that my old dreams of love and family unity were never going to be a reality, and that I needed to take a new direction, starting with the writing course. Katrina had for some time been suggesting I write about my experiences with ovarian cancer and share the positive aspects of my complementary therapies. My decision to pursue this in conjunction with the TAFE course made her happy. We shared a big, warm hug.

My interview with the tutor went well, and she was happy to accept my completed year at Boxhill TAFE in 1994, making me eligible to do her subject of Non Fiction Project, Year 2. She was a very warm lady who said she felt drawn to me, and we parted affectionately.

When I next saw my physician, he listened to my reasons for discontinuing chemotherapy, and then reminded me how it worked. Although the first two sessions killed a lot of the cancer cells, it would only be a short time before they recovered, and re-divided with a vengeance. He suggested it might be wiser to have at least two more sessions rather than to have gone through all that I had for such a short-term result. This gave me food for thought.

Feeling on a high, I bought myself a meal of Thai sweet and sour prawns for tea, and fell asleep that night feeling happier and more content than I had for a long time. The realization and acceptance that nobody had a perfect family, and we were all individuals on our own journeys, and that I would continue to enjoy the happy times when we came together, but accept the reality and limitations within my extended family, gave me peace. As for feeling incomplete without a special someone, it was more important that I loved myself for who I was, and not waste time longing for something I had no control over.

Katrina rang early the next day to say she'd call in for a cuppa and news on her way into Wangaratta. We chatted happily for half an hour, and she left Alex with me while she went shopping. I rang my physician with the decision to go on with chemo, but said I would like better nausea control if possible. I also rang Mum with the news about TAFE and chemo, and spoke to Bren who happened to be there. Pauline called in later in the day, and she was happy that I had found my reason to go on.

The following week was spent happily enjoying day-to-day living, including time with the boys, and social interactions with friends.

On my first day at TAFE, there were eight of us in the class, varying in age, and I was the oldest. They were an extrovert and lively lot, most of them already knowing each other from the previous year. We each spoke about the proposed subject for our project, and the general opinion was that no one would buy a book about ovarian cancer, and that I should concentrate on newspaper and magazine articles.

But that was not what I wanted to do. I was not ready to tell them that I was writing from personal experience, as I wanted honest feedback, and not have them just being nice to me because I had cancer.

Doubts flooded my mind. Was my experience so unique that the general public would want to read about it? Could I make a difference to women's awareness of early symptoms, and alert doctors and make them more curious? I felt I didn't really fit into the class mould. I wasn't working for a diploma and a future job as the majority of the other students were; I was having a race with time. Did it matter if it wasn't commercial, or did Katrina just want it as a memory of her mother? Was that enough reason to do it?

Meantime, I had an assignment to think about, an interview with a published non-fiction author, and I had just the right person in mind, a fellow walker.

The following weekend was the one in which the walking group was staying at the Wangaratta Ski Lodge at Mt St Bernard and doing some alpine walks. I would go armed with pen and paper and hope for an opportunity to interview Adrian while we were there.

I travelled to the Alps with Ivan and Lois, and our arrival coincided with most of the participants. We all settled into our rooms before relaxing for 'happy hour' and to discuss the weekend program.

A thick fog shrouded the lodge in the morning, so it was decided to drive to the other side of the range, where past experience had shown the fog might have cleared. As I was feeling below par, I - with two others - decided against going. I enjoyed a quiet day reading, with a gentle stroll in the vicinity of the lodge when the fog lifted after lunch. The walkers returned footsore and weary late afternoon, and I had the opportunity to interview Adrian during 'happy hour' that evening.

I was feeling rested and refreshed on the Sunday, and enjoyed a not too strenuous walk with the group in the morning, before we packed up and returned home. It had been a great weekend of comradeship, making me feel more 'normal'.

I was due to see the oncologist the following day for blood test results and to arrange further chemo. My blood cells were back to normal, and my CA-125 was down to 17! I received numerous phone calls wishing me well for the next day.

Immediately before my third dose of chemo, I was given the added drugs to try to control my anxiety and nausea (Atavan and Serenace). They made me feel very drowsy, and the oncology nurse was quite concerned. Katrina supported me to her car and drove me home when the chemo was completed. I still vomited, but had the added inconvenience of being sleepy and very shaky on my feet.

The next three days were a daze of giddiness, nausea and vomiting, during which I struggled unsuccessfully to remain hydrated. The oncology nurse had told me I was welcome to come in for more IV fluids if I needed them, so on the Friday, Pauline dropped me off at the oncology ward for a couple of hours while she attended her U3A class. Two litres of IV fluid had me feeling like a new woman.

I slowly improved during the next few days as I was able tolerate food again. Sleep evaded me, and I was still shaky at times, but I had minimal trouble with headaches.

I managed some time with the boys, and was playing with them in the sandpit when Thomas said, "We have to look after you Grandma. The best we can do is keep you well so you don't die."

I guessed he was quoting Lesley, so I made light of it and changed the subject. It was never mentioned again.

I typed up my TAFE assignment over the weekend. The interview had helped clarify in my mind the form my book would take.

I was still feeling below par and shaky at times on Monday, so I rang the oncology nurse for advice. She suggested another litre of IV fluid might help, so Katrina dropped me off at the hospital in the afternoon while she did her shopping, and I did feel stronger afterwards. I hadn't lost my hair but it was thinning as before, but not to the extent that anyone else would notice, and I was most relieved. Perhaps the fresh fruit and vegetable juices and anti-oxidant tablets had helped again. Meantime, a corner had broken off one of my molars and part of the filling fell out. The dentist smoothed the sharp edge, but wouldn't refill it while I was undergoing chemotherapy.

My second class at TAFE was more positive. I hadn't missed any tuition the previous week as students had taken it in turns talking about their book proposals, answering questions and receiving feedback to test their viability. When my turn came, I decided to reveal my state of health in relation to my project, and I received positive support from the class, and the compliment from the tutor that 'My enthusiasm, combined with my intellect were my greatest assets." During the break, I chatted with my fellow students and got to know some a little better.

A backward step

Two weeks after my chemo session when I was expecting to be feeling stronger, my health started deteriorating. I became bloated and nauseated and couldn't face food.

I had arranged to participate in a gentle walk along the Murray River adjacent to St Leonard's winery with the walking group on the Sunday, and although feeling below par, decided to go anyway. Not a good decision.

I had not gone far when dizziness overcame me and I had to rest while the others went on. I managed to eat and drink a little and made it back to the cars, and was very glad to get home. I collapsed into my chair feeling exhausted and shaky.

I had planned a trip the next day to visit Mum then on to see Samantha for her second birthday, but realised I was in no fit state to be driving long distances, so rang to cancel arrangements. I took my temperature on retiring and found it was elevated.

I developed diarrhoea the next morning, so rang the oncology nurse to see if I could come in and see a doctor. Katrina drove me in, and although I was unable to see my own physician, the registrar on duty was most kind and thorough and wanted to admit me into a ward. I declined, as I didn't want to be exposed to the possibility of infection while my immunity was so low. My blood pressure was only 100 over 60. The nurse had difficulty finding a vein, and after taking blood for pathology, gave me a litre of IV fluid, which made me feel a little better.

I rested for the remainder of the day once I was home again, and felt a little better by the next morning.

My recovery was short-lived and I was feeling weak and clammy when the day dawned for my appointment with the oncologist prior to my next chemo session. She read the pathology results and told me that my platelet and white cell counts were dangerously low, too low to have chemo the following week. She still wanted me to have at least one more session when my blood count was near normal again.

Meanwhile, I was to have another blood test the following day and ring her for the result the day after that. If the cells had not recovered sufficiently, I was to have a transfusion of platelets as I was running the risk of spontaneous haemorrhage.

I left her office feeling stunned, and cursing chemotherapy.

My platelet count had improved marginally, sufficient to avoid the transfusion, but I had a long way to go to be back to normal. I spent the next few days quietly at home, and received flowers and encouraging messages from family and friends.

I had another blood test four days later. My oncologist called me with the result, the CA-125 was 11, and the other tests much improved. Although she was still keen for me to have more chemotherapy, she explained that she would have to reduce the dose because of my reaction to it, making it not worth having. I then told her I was going to refuse further treatment regardless, as I had fulfilled the required criterion of two negative CA-125 results, meaning the chemo had done all it could at that stage.

Her final message to me was that if the cancer became active again within six months, I would need to try a different drug regime, but if it was over six months, the same drugs could be repeated. I didn't even want to think that far ahead. I just wanted to celebrate the end of this chemotherapy treatment and get well and strong again.

My physician would later describe my reaction as 'chemo poisoning', and that was certainly how it felt, and I resolved there and then never to subject my body to chemotherapy again, no matter what.

Many months later I found out that the cluster headaches I had experienced were a common side effect of the anti-nausea drug I was having; why hadn't my physician or oncologist picked that up?

On the 16th of March, I put pen to paper and started writing and researching my book.

On the 21st of that same month, my fourth grandchild was born; a healthy baby boy Greg and Jane named Mathew. I couldn't wait to go down to see them all and cuddle the little darling, my reward for going through chemo again.

In August, my CA125 started rising again.

Peace

Sunday 1st September 2002.

I have just been for a walk along my road, to ease the kinks out of my body after a day writing.

It's been a perfect day to herald the start of spring; azure sky with a few puffs of cloud to the south, suggesting a change might be on the way.

The sounds I heard were pure country; the occasional lowing of cattle and the urgent bleat of a ewe as she called her lambs to suckle; the rattle of willy wagtails and the musical twitter of the wrens; the occasional caw of a distant crow, and the melodic carol of a magpie.

Rugged Mt Buffallo was silhouetted on the horizon, and in the distance, brilliant white snowcaps glistened on the highest peaks of the Alps.

The hum of bees as they attended the nodding hellebors and golden daffodils filled my ears as I re-entered my garden. From her place in the sun, Megan arose to rub a friendly greeting around my legs.

How could I feel anything but peace in this setting, even with the knowledge that this could be my final spring in this life?

Whatever happens, I will face each hurdle as it comes with all the courage I can muster, and keep the statisticians busy re-writing.

Epilogue

By January 2003, my CA-125 had risen to 542, and my physician urged me to consider further treatment. To my mind, further chemotherapy was out of the question.

I was feeling tired and had a 'niggle' in the region of my liver, but CT scans and plain x-rays all came up negative.

Armed with these, I went to consult my gyn/oncologist in Melbourne in early February. It was so lovely to see her again, and I congratulated her on becoming a mother again since we had last met.

She perused the films and reports and suggested I have a PET scan, a relatively new diagnostic test not as yet available in regional areas of Victoria. It is similar to a CT scan, but takes closer 'slices', showing up smaller lesions.

She arranged this for the following week. It was more involved than a CT scan and fairly unpleasant, but not too bad. Yet another CT scan followed the PET scan.

The results revealed a small lesion between my liver and diaphragm, and my gyn/oncologist consulted with a radiotherapy team at Peter McCallum Cancer Institute in East Melbourne about the feasibility of treatment.

As it was the only lesion visible in my whole body, it was decided to treat it aggressively with the aim of eliminating it, hopefully putting me once more in remission. I had a very positive feeling that this would be the end of my disease, so agreed to undergoing radiotherapy.

As it was crucial that the lesion be radiated while

still small, arrangements were made very rapidly, and I was scheduled for six weeks of intensive radiotherapy commencing on the last day of March 2003.

Two weeks before commencement of treatment, I had to attend Peter Mc for 'simulation'. This was necessary to determine the treatment area, and enable marks to be tattooed on my skin to assist accurate positioning during treatment. Lying perfectly still on a hard metal table with my arms above my head for and hour or so was the most uncomfortable part of the whole treatment process, and I have four little green tattoo spots as a souvenir for the rest of my life.

I also attended the Familial Cancer Centre adjacent to the hospital to discuss genetic testing. My DNA was accepted for genetic testing and I await the results. *(See Appendix 7, 'Hope for a future - latest research')*

Katrina and I travelled to Melbourne the day before treatment was to commence, and she helped me move into the very comfortable apartments Peter Mc has close to the hospital, and stayed with me for the first few days. Another set of x-rays to confirm alignment, and I was ready to commence radiotherapy the following day.

Fear of the unknown was the worst aspect, but I soon settled into a routine of treatment and recreation, supported by a wonderful team of doctors, nurses, dietitians, social workers and volunteers, plus family and friends, all intent on making it as positive an experience as possible.

Mothers' Day fell during the time I was in Melbourne, and as weekends were treatment-free, I travelled to Healesville by public transport to visit my mother. Brenda picked me up from the bus and I stayed overnight at her home.

After spending time with Mum, Brenda and I took the dogs for a walk through the bushland we both loved adjacent to her home. We were relaxed and comfortable together, and all past differences seemed to evaporate into insignificance. We parted with a warm and sincere hug. This feeling of closeness has continued and brought me great peace.

I was fortunate and did not experience extreme side effects during treatment, but was very tired by the end of the six weeks, and grateful to be back in the comfort, peace and quiet of my own home, and the welcoming company of my cat.

A blood test a week later showed my CA-125 down to 36, but my white cell count was also down, leaving me vulnerable to infection, and as a consequence, I picked up a virus, which developed into bronchitis. By late June 2003, my CA-125 was 20.

Time has slowly but surely healed my relationship with Rob, and I was once more included as part of the team during the busy hay season of 2003, which added greatly to the quality and happiness of my life.

With another phase of my disease and treatment behind me, I am feeling great. I'm getting on with my life with huge hopes for a long and healthy future, boxing gloves at the ready.

'No *coward soul is mine,*
No trembler in the world's storm-troubled sphere:
I see heaven's glories shine,
And faith shines equal, arming me from fear.'

Emily Brontë.

Appendix 1

What is Ovarian Cancer?

Ovarian Cancer is the general term for cancer originating in the ovary, and can be of three types – epithelial cancer, germ cell tumors, and specialized stromal cell cancers. The three types of cells that the ovaries are made up of are the bases for the three types of cancer that occur. About 80% of ovarian cancers are epithelial, 20% germ cell, and what little is left are specialized stromal cell cancers.

Cells from other cancers such as breast or intestinal cancers, can metastasize or spread to the ovary, and are referred to as Krukenberg tumors.

The majority of women who have ovarian cancer will have to deal with epithelial cancer, of which there are seven types, however symptoms and treatment are similar. What is more important to understand are the stages.

Surgical stages of Ovarian Cancer

Stage 1 — Limited to the ovaries.

- 1A — One ovary involved (contained)
- 1B — Both ovaries involved.
- 1C — One or both ovaries involved, but with cancer on the surface of an ovary, rupture of an ovarian cyst, malignant ascites (fluid in the abdominal cavity) or positive abdominal washings (fluid from the abdomen is checked under the microscope for signs of cancer).

Stage	2	Spread to adjacent pelvic structures.
	2A	Spread to uterus or fallopian tubes.
	2B	Spread to pelvic peritoneum.
	2C	Confined to the pelvis, but with malignant ascites or positive abdominal washings.
Stage	3	Spread to the upper abdomen.
	3A	Microscopic spread to the upper abdomen
	3B	Cancer nodules less than 2 cm in the abdomen.
	3C	Nodules more than 2 cm, or positive pelvic or aortic lymph nodes.
Stage 4		Distant spread beyond the abdomen, liver, lung, etc. This stage is determined at surgery.

No matter how good and thorough your surgeon is, there is often some cancer remaining, except in the earliest stages. A good surgeon, or a gyn/oncologist, a surgeon who specialises in cancer of the reproductive system, is your best choice, and will remove any nodules larger than 1 cm (1/4 inch). This may necessitate the removal of a piece of intestine, which will be re-joined, or a colostomy formed (an opening onto the abdomen).

The Grade of the Cancer Cells

The grade is as important as the stage, and determines to a large degree, the on-going treatment. The grade has to do with the behavior of the cancers, meaning how quickly or slowly they grow, and is judged by the appearance of the cells under the microscope.

Well-differentiated cancers, in which clear types of cells grow, tend to grow and spread more slowly. On the other hand, cancers with undifferentiated cells tend to grow and spread more quickly.

- Borderline – Grade 0 – grows and spreads slowly.
- Well-differentiated – Grade 1 – grows and spreads a little more quickly.
- Moderately differentiated – Grade 2 – grows and spreads rapidly.
- Poorly or undifferentiated – Grade 3 – grows and spreads very rapidly.

Armed with this information, a woman with ovarian cancer may choose to ask her physician or oncologist what type, stage and grade her ovarian cancer is, and have a little more idea what he/she is talking about.

Treatment

Borderline cancers, that is, epithelial ovarian cancer of low malignant potential, based on microscopic appearance, are not usually treated further as they are very slow growing. Signs of re-growth may occur in 15-20 years, but most never recur.

The initial treatment of epithelial ovarian cancer is the surgical removal of the uterus, fallopian tubes, ovaries, and any large nodules of cancer. An exception is made if the woman is still of childbearing age and wishes to have more children, and the cancer is confined to one ovary. She is strongly advised to have the remaining ovary removed at a later stage. Chemotherapy usually follows the removal of the affected ovary.

It is seldom all the cancer can be removed, but if no nodules larger than 1-2 cm remain, that is considered optimal. After surgery, almost all patients will require further treatment.

Always remember, it is **your** choice of when and what treatment you choose to have or not have. Your greatest weapon is information, so always go to the oncologist or physician armed with a note pad of questions, and write down the answers as you get them, and/or have someone with you, or a tape recorder to jolt your memory. You will probably be in an emotional turmoil, and physically below par, and cannot be expected to have total recall.

Most importantly, you are the expert when it comes to how you are feeling, physically, emotionally and spiritually.

As suggested by Arlene Cotter in her book *From this Moment On,* 'If you are confused and uncertain, you might like to get someone you trust to ask you the following questions, and either vocalize or write down your responses. Your answers may change at different stages of your disease and treatment.'

- What is your body telling you?
- What beliefs do you have about what has happened to you?
- How strong is your will?
- What do you want to happen next?'

APPENDIX 2
Treatment Choices

After surgery for ovarian cancer, you basically have four treatment choices:

1. Chemotherapy and/or radiation therapy. Chemotherapy can also be given before surgery.
2. Alternative therapies.
3. A combination of alternative therapy and chemotherapy (holistic medicine).
4. 'Wait and see', where your physician closely monitors your symptoms.

Some women may not need chemotherapy because their cancer was either not aggressive or it was caught at an early stage, and the chances are extremely high that they will not have a recurrence.

Chemotherapy.

Often shortened to 'chemo', it merely means 'drug treatment'. It can be given via IV (intravenously i.e. directly into the bloodstream via a needle in the vein), orally (by mouth), or IP (directly into the peritoneal cavity via a plastic tube through the abdominal wall).

Radiation was not usually used for ovarian cancer because of the major side effects, and the fact that chemo works so well, as a rule.

Chemotherapy is commenced soon after surgery, and is usually repeated every 3-4 weeks for an average of six sessions. A combination of two or more drugs is usual in order to produce the best possible response to treatment. I have not been able to find out exactly why different patients are given different drug combinations, but I expect it depends on the type of epithelial cancer, and the stage and grade, as well as the patient's age and overall health at the time. This could be a good question to ask your oncologist.

'Remember that the human body is tough and strong, and that cancer cells are not invincible. Very frequently, cancer cells are so weak and vulnerable that they die by the millions when exposed to chemotherapy drugs. Your body is a more complex organism than cancer, and that you can help give yourself the strength to weather a chemical storm'
From *Making the Chemotherapy Decision* by David Drum.

How do you know if it's working?

- If there is a visible or measurable cancer (on CT scan or ultrasound), and it has reduced in size.
- If ascites (fluid in the abdominal cavity) has been present before and has not recurred.
- If the CA-125 was elevated and reverts to normal (below 15).

Radiation Therapy

Also known as radiotherapy, this has not been a common option in OVCA until recently. Considerable research and pioneering has been taking place at Peter MacCallum Cancer Institute in East Melbourne by a dedicated team of radiation oncologists, enabling some specific cases of OVCA where there is an isolated lesion, to be treated with radiotherapy.

Alternative Therapies

There are a lot of choices out there, so talk to naturopaths, search the web, talk to fellow cancer patients, and read, read, read. I am convinced that Mother Nature provides a cure for everything that can ail us, it's just a matter of finding it. I also believe in the power of mind over matter.

Positive thinking and having an important reason to go on living are major factors, and having emotional support is imperative. **This does not mean that if you don't survive you have failed in any way.** We can each only do our best, knowing the true secrets of our hearts and minds, and it's for no one else to judge.

The combination of alternative therapy and chemotherapy

This is the road I have taken, and it has been the right decision for me. The thought of chemotherapy drugs invading my body is still loathsome, but I know they have prolonged my life. I also believe that the complementary therapies I have implemented have added to my time.

I am convinced that stress is the greatest enemy of people fighting cancer, but who in this life can be completely immune and sheltered from the highs and lows of day to day living? The fact that we all react differently to stress is a contributing factor, and how we feel emotionally, physically and spiritually supported.

Through experience, I believe that meditation can contribute immensely to the management of stress and the maintenance of peace and well-being.

The wait and see policy

During this time, your physician closely monitors you. This is an option I have taken when free of symptoms, while my CA-125 climbed. I was unwilling to deliberately make myself sick with chemo, and undermine my quality of life before I had to. The disadvantage of this option is that you're never sure if any little incident of pain or discomfort is the cancer at work, an everyday twinge experienced by most people, or your hyperactive imagination.

Only you can decide which path to take, at which period of your disease and treatment. There is no right or wrong way.

Appendix 3
How Chemotherapy Works

To understand how chemotherapy works, it is necessary to understand the nature of cancer cells. Cancers are thought to arise as a single cell, and it is the abnormal multiplication of this cell as it divides uncontrollably that forms a cancer.

Normal cells divide only enough to replace those that are lost, or to replace injury such as a cut finger or broken bone, then stop dividing, but cancer cells have lost this restraint and keep dividing. The mass of cancer cells will eventually become large enough to cause problems. This will produce a lump, mass or tumor that can be detected. ('Oncology' means the study of lumps.)

This mass of cancer cells has to have a blood supply, so it causes neighboring blood cells to grow into it. These blood vessels are often faulty and break easily, therefore bleeding is often one of the signs of cancer. They are also poor in carrying blood and oxygen, so the mass of cancer cells can be relatively oxygen deficient making them vulnerable to decay, which is why some cancers have an odor. The mass of cancer cells has the ability to invade into adjacent tissue and spread to distant sites (metastasise).

Cancers cause problems because they grow and occupy space, pushing on other structures causing them to malfunction. They have no nerve supply so they do not hurt, but they can cause pain in other structures because of the destruction and pressure. Cancers need energy to grow and rob the body of energy it needs for normal function.

The aim of chemotherapy is to kill off the cancer cells, allowing the normal cells to recover and resume normal function.

Because cancer cells grow and increase more quickly than normal cells, the theory is that they will absorb more of the chemotherapy drugs than the normal cells and be killed off more quickly.

When cancer is active, not all the cells are at the same stage of maturity. The first dose of chemo knocks out the mature cells that are present at that time. When the second dose of chemo is given, say in 2-3 weeks time, a further lot of cells have matured, and these are knocked out. Thus it proceeds with the ongoing chemotherapy sessions until there are a negligible number of active cells surviving, and these are considered too weak to multiply.

The normal cells have a 'memory', and this is triggered to recover and re-grow the normal cells e.g. blood cells, between treatments. The cells in all parts of the body, excluding the brain and spinal column, are continually dying and being replaced, but at differing rates depending on the organ in question. The rate at which cells normally die and are replaced dictates the side affects, for example, hair grows quickly, so the hair follicles are severely affected, leading to hair loss, and likewise, the cells lining the stomach, causing the nausea commonly experienced.

With ovarian cancer, the usual rule of thumb is that if there are two consecutive negative CA-125 results, the chemotherapy is thought to have done all it can at that stage.

Appendix 4
Second Look Surgery

Laparotomy is the medical term for 'incising the abdominal wall for exploratory purposes'. second look surgery is a major operation. The surgeon thoroughly explores and biopsies every organ in the abdominal cavity, and sometimes removes all the lymphatic glands in there as well. It may be performed regardless of the fact that X-rays, CT scans, CA-125 and physical examinations are all normal.

If no more cancer is found, then nothing needs to be done, but the patient still has to recover from the operation. This carries the risk of infection and complications, and on-going oedema (swelling due to excess fluid in the tissues, especially affecting the legs) if the glands have been removed, which can be painful and debilitating.

If cancer is detected, more treatment needs to be given. But here is the dilemma. The best known treatment has already been given, and the odds are poor that any other treatment will be effective.

If the second look is negative, the odds of cancer recurring are still 50%.

If you and your surgeon are contemplating second look surgery, you must have a clear idea why you are doing it and what you are going to do with the results. Ask questions, and don't be bullied into a decision because 'it's normal procedure'.

It's your body and your life they are dealing with!

Appendix 5

Journey's End – a guide for patients and carers

What if treatment is no longer working?

Most patients with ovarian cancer do well after initial treatment, for varying lengths of time, but few will be cured (about 15%). For them, and their families and friends, it will be an emotional roller coaster of fear and hope. Life seems to evolve around the CA-125 results and decisions about treatment. This is when it is of utmost importance to live one day at a time, and concentrate on the good things in life.

When ovarian cancer persists despite several different treatments and regimes, it's time to make a decision on overall goals. Cure is seldom a realistic goal, but for some, anything else is untenable. Major cancer treatment centres offer a range of extreme treatments such as high-dose chemotherapy, bone marrow and stem cell replacement and gene therapy. Ask your oncologist for details. Miracles are also sought through alternate therapies in various places around the world. It's up to you.

A more realistic goal, for me anyway, is learning to live with the cancer, knowing that you will die of it some day, BUT YOU ARE NOT DEAD YET. As Dr. Bernie Siegal said, 'No one ever died of statistics.'

Use this time to do what is important to you. For some it is a concerted effort to fulfill dreams and goals. Make a list if you like, and put it in order of priority, and go for it. This is not a time to be shy about asking favors.

I have found that family and friends are more than happy to be involved in such positive activity rather than waiting around doing nothing until you die. I'm still aiming for a flight in a Tiger Moth, tandem hang gliding, a flight over Antarctica, and seeing whales close up.

Resolve those issues with other people that are still troubling you. If you are unable to do it face-to-face for some reason, imagine them sitting opposite you and have a conversation with them, saying all that needs to be said, then ask for understanding/forgiveness. Most importantly, forgive yourself.

Writing down everything you need and want to say to someone can also be therapeutic. The recipient need never read it; sometimes it's better if it isn't. The important thing is to get it out of your system. I have found burning the paper in a flowerpot outside and watching the smoke float away with the conflict, most therapeutic.

If there are special people in your life you want to spend time with saying goodbye, make the time, and enjoy the moment. Write letters and make tapes to be read or heard on significant occasions in the future, if that will give you peace. I am writing individual letters to my grandchildren to be opened on their 18th birthdays. I am also recording the children's stories I have written so they can hear me reading to them. As I have mentioned, when I first came out of remission, I had studio photos taken, and had the best of them framed as gifts to my family; I want to be remembered with my hair on!

Make peace with your God if you have one, and know that he/she loves you unconditionally.

'Yesterday is history; tomorrow a mystery; but today is a gift –that is why it is called the present.' (*Source unknown*)

If you haven't already done so, make or update your will. It is also most helpful if you have available a list of bank accounts, DSS number if applicable, funeral fund details, and all those other day-to-day details your next of kin will have to deal with. I have made a list additional to my will, of things I would like particular people to have, and have put a sticker with their name inconspicuously on the article, where possible. I have made it clear to my children that it is their choice whether they follow this through or not.

You might like to make it known to those concerned what form you would like your funeral to take, remembering that legally, what becomes of your earthly remains is entirely up to your next of kin. I know someone who has already written her form of service, and selected the speakers and music, and written her own eulogy. I wouldn't go that far, practical as I am, but I hope to find the time to record the list of my favorite music and why I like it.

Palliative Care

As I have been in the position of nurse, volunteer and recipient of palliative care, I feel I can speak with authority on this delicate subject. I say delicate, as I am all too aware that the term palliative can have a negative impact, and I would like to somehow make it more 'user-friendly'.

Having completed the training course in palliative care as a registered nurse, I knew of the value and expertise this knowledge lends to the care and comfort of patients with life threatening illness. But when I was approached post-operatively by a palliative care representative, my reaction was totally negative, and I made it quite clear that I didn't consider myself in need of their services, and wouldn't be for some time.

Mine was not an unusual reaction as I learnt later when training as a palliative care volunteer. Even some doctors are reluctant to suggest the service to their patients in fear of upsetting them.

So what is it about the title 'palliative' that evokes such a negative response?

'Palliate' means to alleviate (disease) without curing, recognising that at some point of a person's illness there is a change from a curative focus to that of controlling and alleviating symptoms.

Palliative care aims to make a person feel in control of their treatment and their quality of life by treating their symptoms to make them more comfortable. This is achieved by controlling their pain and helping them make changes that will make their life easier.

This positive aspect seems to be overwhelmed by the attitude that if a patient is eligible for palliative care they are 'doomed'.

As a recipient of palliative care while I was undergoing my second course of chemotherapy, I found the service and staff positive and caring, and was most grateful for their concern and attention to both Katrina and myself. When I was well again the service was withdrawn, but if and when I need it again I will be happy to use it, and be grateful for its existence.

The philosophy and object of palliative care are summarised in the words of Dame Cicely Saunders, founder of St Christopher's Hospice.

"You matter because you are you.
You matter to the last moment of your life,
And we will do all we can,
Not only to help you die in peace,
But also to live until you die."

The official objectives as cited by the Palliative Care Council and the Victorian Palliative Care Education and

Training Committee, 1989, in a report to the Minister for Health Victoria, are based on meeting the physical and emotional needs of terminally ill people; reducing or preventing pain and other symptoms; offering support to the patients family and caregivers; giving a choice with respect to the site of care; and providing bereavement counselling.

The palliative care service.

Palliative care can be provided in the person's home, at a specialist in-patient hospice, or at some other health facility, depending on where the person is living and where they choose to die, and complements the range of medical treatments and services already available.

Each palliative care service provides its own program of services to the person and their family. This may include nursing, medical consultancy, day care, counselling, diet advice, loan of equipment, physiotherapy, occupational therapy, social worker services, bereavement support, pastoral care, and a wide range of support from trained volunteers.

You can be referred to the service by anyone who is caring for you, including health professionals, your family and friends, or you can refer yourself, and it is available for all people facing life-threatening illness.

The provision of palliative care relies on commonwealth and state government funding, so palliative care is generally free. However, most community based palliative care services are charitable organisations that rely on donations and fundraising to supplement the funds they receive. Hospitals and hospices may charge fees for in-patients, but Medicare or private insurance usually covers these fees. There may be a charge for the hire of some equipment. Medication and supplies are purchased in the usual way.

Pain relief.

Most people's greatest fear when they face a terminal disease, is of the pain they may suffer towards the end. I certainly fit into this category.

In almost all cases, pain can be overcome or made quite tolerable: in all cases it can be eased to some degree. It is important to realise that although pain occurs in many life-threatening illnesses, not everyone will experience it. It is very important for you to be able to speak openly about pain and discomfort and to ask your doctor or nurse any question that is on your mind. Here are some things you may want to know about pain control.

Opioids are a family of drugs used to relieve pain and other symptoms such as breathlessness. Morphine is one of the best-known and most commonly used opioid. There are many myths about morphine and its use, and unreasonable fear of using morphine sometimes leads people to conceal their pain or refuse medication. This can cause unnecessary suffering to both the person and their family.

Here are some of the facts about morphine:

- Morphine and other opioids are not psychologically addictive when properly prescribed for pain relief.
- Morphine is often prescribed early in the course of an illness in order to manage pain. This is not a sign that death is close. People taking morphine to control pain may be able to live normally, going about their lives in the usual way. Using morphine to control pain may mean that the person can continue to go to work, drive a car, go on holiday, go to special family events and enjoy life largely free of pain.

- Properly prescribed, morphine will not hasten death. It can improve the quality and length of remaining life.
- No two people are the same. Dose requirements for morphine vary enormously. One person may need only 5 milligrams to control pain, another, 500 milligrams or more. Only the individual can tell when the pain is eased.
- Morphine can be given in many forms including oral mixtures, tablets or injections.
- Opioids have side effects. Constipation is to be expected and is controlled by diet and laxatives. Any initial drowsiness and nausea usually clears up in a few days. They can be eased by other medication, or controlled by changing the dose or formulation. Other side affects are rare.
- Not everyone with a life-threatening illness or cancer has to take morphine.
- People are sometimes concerned that if they use morphine to control pain early in their illness there may be no other way to control pain if it increases later on. This is not so. The appropriate doses will, in almost all cases, continue to relieve pain right through the course of the illness.

General pain relief.

Each person is different. Keep your doctor or visiting nurse fully informed about any pain you are experiencing so that they can:

- Select the right medication, ranging from paracetamol to morphine.
- Start the pain relief in good time and increase the dose, or move to a more powerful drug as the pain increases.

- Give you regular doses to keep the pain at bay. It is better to take pain medication regularly to prevent pain rather than to let the pain return and then relieve it.

By discussing your medication with your doctor or visiting nurse you will be helping to control the pain, not allowing the pain to control you.

Other medications including anti-arthritic drugs, muscle relaxants, and anti-depressants also help to relieve pain in some cases.

Cancer pain can also be relieved through radiotherapy, or chemotherapy by tablets or injections. These treatments aim to relieve pain by killing cancer cells and stopping growth of tumors.

While medication is important in controlling pain, many other methods make a contribution. These include massage, meditation, relaxation training, psychotherapy and support groups, as well as other complementary treatments.

Your doctor or visiting nurse will find the pain relief that suits you best.

Palliative care recognises that there is not only physical pain, but there can be emotional and/or spiritual pain too. There are staff and volunteers in palliative care services who have a special interest in spiritual issues, and so can help both you and your family.

Closeness and touch from people you love are important for you and for them. This is a time when people who are close can give their greatest support by expressing their love and their feelings openly and saying their good-byes.

The patient's right.

Your rights, including your right to refuse treatment, are set out under various laws. You can also appoint a friend or relative to act on your behalf, should you become incapacitated. The Medical Treatment Act 1988 of Victoria, and equivalent Acts throughout Australia cover these decisions.

If you have concerns, by discussing these matters in advance with your doctor and members of the family, you can ensure that your wishes will be taken into account if and when you are no longer able to make decisions for yourself. You may also want to discuss these matters with your solicitor or social worker.

Be comforted by the motto of the palliative care nursing service:

'To cure sometimes;
To relieve often;
To comfort always.'

End Stage

When the disease has taken charge of the body and death is obviously approaching, it is known as the end stage. Obviously I cannot as yet speak from personal experience, but I have witnessed it numerous times.

My overall impression is that when a person enters this stage, there is generally a peaceful detachment by them from what is going on with his/her body. I have often had the feeling that their spirit is already free and just waiting around for the body to stop functioning completely before they depart this existence.

There will still be lucid times and it is great if these can be shared and enjoyed with loved ones, and I'm sure that during the final process of dying, a patient is more at peace and pain free if in a loving environment. This can be either in their home or that of a loved one, or in a hospice or palliative care unit. I believe that it is those you are with that is important in the end, and not where you are.

Hopefully, if there is conflict or tension within the family, this can be put aside during this special time of parting, and certainly kept away from the bedside. The patient may seem oblivious, but hearing is the last sense to go and although they don't react, they could still be upset.

There is often a degree of restlessness near to the end, and I hope there will be someone there for me, holding my hand and telling me its okay to go, and that they will always love and remember me.

The remaining part of this segment is for those caring for people at the end of their journey on earth, a most difficult task, but a great act of love.

Home care

As the end stage of the disease approaches and the patient needs more constant care, decisions have to be made by the patient and family about how long and where the patient will be cared for.

The best chance of living as normally as possible in spite of illness is at home. Routines chosen, food eaten, visitors and entertainment are more easily catered for in the home than in the confines of a hospital or hospice. There is privacy to behave and react freely in a home environment.

One of the main benefits of helping someone die at home is that it encourages family and friends to be involved in maintaining the best quality of life possible. Families often feel much closer as a result.

The task will never be easy, and circumstances do not

permit everyone to do it. Do not feel guilty if you start and have to change your mind, or if it is just not possible in the first place.

However, it can be one of life's experiences that is rewarding for all concerned in terms of the opportunity for personal growth and the sense of fulfillment achieved, but you will find that your normal routines change dramatically.

Preparing for home care.

If your family has never been one to communicate and co-operate, don't imagine they will suddenly acquire these skills at this time of need. It may bring out the best in some and aggravate hidden hostilities in others, so getting together before the situation becomes critical and assessing the advantages and disadvantages of home care, and being honest about what each person is willing and able to contribute, is vital. This could include close friends of the patient or family who have expressed a desire to help in any way.

It is most important to recognise your limitations and to think about your resources, both people and services, which will give you support.

The reality.

Caring for a dying person means for 24 hours a day. It is therefore a difficult task on your own, and a friend or relative with nursing experience can be a great help, but lack of such a person or experience does not disqualify you. A loving intent and a willingness to access all the professional care and advice available is sufficient.

Your greatest allies will be your **General Practitioner** who will provide ongoing management of your relation's illness and will help co-ordinate other medical and paramedical services as required.

District Nurses/Palliative Care/ Hospice Nurses will visit regularly according to need and provide assistance with medication, hygiene, pressure care, bowel and bladder management, dressings, injections and so on. Sometimes they will visit just to talk about the care. On other occasions, advice and reassurance over the phone will be all that is necessary.

Occupational Therapists are able to advise on changes in the home to make caring easier, such as ramps, rails, items of equipment e.g. commode, wheelchair.

Social Workers can assist in counselling and inform you about other services that might be helpful, and what financial assistance is available.

Chaplains/Ministers of Religion can provide pastoral care, seeking to integrate spiritual concerns with those physical, social and emotional ones, for both the patient and carer.

Palliative Care Volunteers are trained to provide practical and emotional support. It is often beneficial to have someone who is not emotionally involved supporting you and your family.

It is important to know whom to contact in case of an emergency. Make a list and have it by the phone at all times.

Estimates of how long care is likely to be needed are not always accurate, so it is important to pace yourself, giving yourself the best chance to go the full distance. Make the most of offers of support and share the load, allowing you time-out to relax and unwind before returning to the demands of nursing care. If you become exhausted and stressed out making yourself vulnerable to illness, you have defeated the purpose.

Getting Practical

To make things a little easier for all concerned, a few simple changes may need to be made to the home.

- The bed should be accessible from both sides and have a bedside table. Unnecessary furniture should be removed or rearranged to allow space for wheelchair access, nursing procedures and visitors to attend.
- If possible, an outside view to a garden is desirable, as is a phone extension in the bedroom that can be unplugged at rest times.
- Rails and a shower chair in the bath or shower can be most helpful.
- Changing the door in the toilet to swing out instead of in can give extra space for the assistant. Rails and a raised toilet seat are also helpful.
- A comfortable place can be made in the living area so that the patient can be part of daily activities and conversation when they feel up to it. A cordless phone is useful at such times.
- A removable ramp to negotiate steps can make access in and out of the house easier for a wheelchair.
- A simple bell or a remote call system will give the carer more freedom to move around the house and garden, and give the patient more confidence and peace of mind.

Some extra equipment may be required depending on the progress of the disease and the degree of immobility and dependence, and access and proximity to the toilet and bathroom. These may include:

- A special mattress to reduce the risk of pressure areas,
- Sheepskins to sit/sleep on and to protect heels,
- Extra pillows,

- Waterproof mattress protector, special absorbent sheets ('kylies'), or 'blueys' - disposable plastic-backed rectangles to place under the patient's buttocks while sitting or lying,
- A bed table or tray,
- Flexible straws or a feeding mug with a spout,
- A commode, bedpan or bottle,
- Wash basin or shower chair,
- Wheelchair or walking aid,
- A hospital-type bed or reclining chair.

These items can be hired or borrowed from a variety of sources such as district/palliative care nursing services, occupational therapy departments, Red Cross Society or pharmacies.

What to expect.

Following are the more common problems occurring in advanced illness.

Pain. This is a universal fear for cancer patients, but not all suffer pain, but in ovarian cancer, bowel obstruction and/or liver failure are often the final cause of death, and skill and experience on the part of the attending doctors and nurses is needed to keep the patient comfortable.

Pain may be aggravated by emotional and social problems, which may need attention also. Prescribed medication should be taken strictly around the clock, not waiting for pain to return before giving the next dose.

As explained under Palliative Care, morphine is not a last resort, and addiction is not a problem. Other medications may be used with morphine.

Nausea and vomiting. This may be due to a variety of causes, requiring specific medications, which can be given in a number of different ways. Nausea can in fact be more of a problem than vomiting if it lingers. Strong cooking smells and heavily perfumed flowers can aggravate nausea.

Not eating/losing weight. Carers seem to have the universal need to see the patient eat to feel they are doing a good job. Rather than worrying about balanced meals at specific times, encourage patients to eat a little of what they like, when they like, concentrating on foods that are easily digested. High calorie drinks are useful.

Constipation. Inactivity, poor nutrition and fluid intake, dehydration, weakness and drugs make this a common problem. But even with a poor diet, the intestine makes enough faeces for a bowel action about every three days. Encourage mobility, more fluids, and prompt response to the desire to use the bowels. With morphine, treating it in anticipation with laxatives controls constipation. Visiting nurses may need to help with suppositories or enemas. Proper bowel care is essential and is worth disturbing the patient for.

Skin care. The prevention of pressure sores, skin rashes and cracks is most important. Where the body is in constant contact with the bed – heels, hipbones, buttocks, and elbows are the areas most at risk. If the patient is confined to bed frequently, sheepskin, special sheets, bed cradles, thorough drying after washing and the appropriate use of talc and moisture cream are helpful, but frequent (2-4 hourly) changes of position are vital. Further advice is best sought from the attending nurses.

Confusion. Disorientation for time and sometimes place is normal in the very ill and dying. Anxiety may aggravate this with nightmares and vivid daydreams. Just sitting with them and talking quietly and calmly may decrease their fear. Sometimes medication or other medical problems such as a full bladder or bowel are responsible, requiring attention by the doctor or nurse.

Continue to treat the patient as a sane and sensible adult. Avoid restraints, and calm down fears by explanation and reassurance. Medication is sometimes necessary, but as far as possible should be used sparingly.

Weakness. Incurred weakness is often one of the most frustrating symptoms for you and your relative to cope with. There may seem to be less interest in activities as the person's strength to be up and about decreases. Inevitably, more time is spent in a chair or in bed. Rest periods between outings and visitors become very important and must be adhered to.

Dehydration. In the final stages of advanced illness, patients often lose interest in fluids as well as food. This is no reflection on your care. It is important to remember that at the end, dehydration is not disturbing the patient, in fact there are a number of advantages; less secretion to swallow or rattle in the back of the throat, coughing is reduced, vomiting is less likely, and there is less urine to pass. This is nature's way of shutting down body processes. The only disadvantage is dryness in the mouth and this can be controlled using small ice blocks to suck, or moistening the mouth with swabs soaked in water or pineapple juice. Vaseline or lanolin prevents lips from cracking. 'Thrush' in the mouth in the form of white fungal plaques requires prescription medication. I.V. fluids are not necessary.

New Skills

There are a number of new skills you can learn from the district nurse, so don't fumble along being independent and feeling inadequate, as you could hurt both the patient and yourself. Among these skills is learning how to transfer patients from bed to a chair or commode; from a wheelchair to the toilet or into a car; and how to position a patient in bed for pressure care and comfort, while preserving your own back.

There are ways of changing wet or soiled bedding, sponging patients in bed, and positioning pillows for posture and comfort. Sometimes specific skills such as emptying a catheter bag might need to be learnt, along with accurate record keeping of medications.

Being aware of what it might be like to have these things done for you is one of the keys of good nursing care. Try at all times to respect the dignity and modesty of the patient.

Learning to listen, encouraging open and honest communication with the expression of thoughts and feelings is a skill worth developing. People with cancer are often frightened, sad or angry. Talking about these things and talking about dying often helps patients overcome despair and gives them peace and quality of life in what time is left. Don't force your need to talk on them, but try to be open and honest about your feelings. Trying to be 'brave' and strong for them creates a barrier to self-expression.

Sometimes neither patient nor loved ones are able to openly express their thoughts and feelings and just being quietly together in peace and harmony is enough.

Managing medication.

Never rely on memory when administering medication. If the nurse doesn't provide a chart, create your own, listing the name of the medication, the dose, the reason it was given, the time and the date.

A useful aid is the use of a 'dosette', available from pharmacies. This is a box divided into compartments for days of the week and intervals through the day. Medication can be set out a week in advance, making the dosette at once a visual reminder and record of the treatment schedule. If several people are sharing the care, it will avoid any mix-ups in medication.

With progress of the illness towards its terminal stages, medication needs to be constantly reviewed, though medication for pain relief should be constant even if the patient is unable to swallow and is sleeping a lot. The doctor or nurse may arrange for that medication to be given by a different route e.g. rectally or by injection, sometimes using a special infusion pump.

Special problems.

Mental and physical deterioration in the patient calls for a lot of patience. This may be the time you and your loved one or whoever is involved in home care may decide on transfer to a hospice or palliative care unit. It is not an admission of inadequacy or a reason to feel guilty, in fact your relative might be embarrassed at your having to attend to their personal hygiene, and feel more secure with professional care. You can still spend as much time as you want with your relation and participate in their care to the degree you are comfortable with, such as massaging their feet and hands, reading to them, playing their favorite music, bringing special treats, supervising visitors, etc.

If you all decide to try and see it through to the end at home, be aware that the course is sometimes unpredictable, but lack of experience does not mean you cannot help. Take each day, one at a time. You will be surprised how much you learn in a short space of time. You probably know more about your relative than anybody else, so you can guide others in their care, including the doctors and nurses, by reminding them of the patient's likes and dislikes.

You can expect it will probably be necessary to help your relative with personal hygiene including assistance passing urine and emptying their bowels. Commodes are generally easier to use than bedpans.

Attention to preventing falls needs to be given by removing floor rugs and using some sort of walking frame. This will give the person more confidence and independence and save your back. With increasing weakness, a wheelchair may become necessary, until finally your relative is confined to bed.

Mental changes can also occur. Sometimes a little or no response may make normal interaction impossible. This can fluctuate hour-to-hour, day-to-day. Confusion and inability to communicate properly makes it difficult to share memories, and missing the kind of relationship established over many years or a lifetime is one of the most stressful aspects of caring for a dying relative. This is the beginning of your loss.

Problems for the Carer.

Many people find that they have to put their lives on hold once they commit themselves to care for a dying relative. Personal, family and professional plans are not made, altered, postponed or dropped altogether. You may be torn between your own family and your dying relative, which could add pressure to an already fragile relationship. There may be a feeling of isolation from family and friends, and as time goes on you may need to regain a balance between caring, and resuming some outside activities.

Personal health may suffer. Tiredness is a common complaint caused not just by lack of sleep, but constant tension and grief. Other people may not recognise the extent of care you are providing when your dying relative rallies while visitors are there. Sometimes carers become the target for patient's feelings.

Another difficulty may be dealing with advice from others unable or unwilling to be directly involved in care, particularly if they are at a different stage of accepting your relative's illness. Handling visitors who stay too long and are insensitive to the patients needs might be another issue.

Keeping a journal of events, your care and feelings, is one way of dealing with those problems yourself, and acts as a safety valve.

It's okay not to cope.

Like the majority of people, you are probably in a situation you have never been in before. Check that you have been looking after yourself by eating regularly and getting enough sleep. Ask yourself when you last did something just for fun such as seeing a movie or going on a picnic, or told someone close to you how you feel.

Mixed feelings are not unusual. You may be feeling grief in anticipation, yet secretly wishing it were all over. You may be almost afraid to leave the bedside for fear of your relative suffering unnecessary discomfort, yet be feeling impatient and frustrated. You may also have a fear that your relative might die while you are away. My experience is that many people choose a time when they are alone to die, so the absence you need may also be their opportunity.

Try not to be too critical of yourself, and take every opportunity you can to talk about your feelings. It may be appropriate to either organise someone else to care for your relative for a while or to arrange respite care in a hospital or hospice for a few days, or a week or so.

Should children be involved?

Children who are involved are more likely to be able to discuss their feelings about illness and death and understand your own commitment. At the same time, do not burden children with adult responsibility, and try to maintain the child's routine and try not to separate family members.

Children can be part of the caring team by doing drawings or writing stories, picking flowers, and talking about their daily activities. Their very presence with its innocence and unconditional love can be enough to brighten the patient's day.

Common sense should prevail to shield them from witnessing their beloved relative suffering pain or vomiting, but they should be aware of what is happening, the degree depending on their age and emotional maturity. Helping to paint the coffin or writing or drawing messages to go in the coffin may be ways you might like children to participate in the actual death.

If a family grieves together, they heal together.

Last minute matters.

Before physical and mental deterioration occurs, it makes life much easier for surviving relations if some of the following are dealt with if not already done.

- The will should be finalised and up to date with circumstances, including the distribution of special belongings.
- Financial arrangements should be such that surviving relatives have access to bank accounts for ongoing expenses.

- Consideration should be given to someone having enduring power of attorney. That person, not necessarily a relative, is able to act in all matters, personal and financial, and make medical decisions should the patient be unable to do so.
- It may be appropriate to talk about the funeral service and whether burial or cremation is preferred.
- Any unresolved issues in your relative's life are best dealt with before it's too late.
- Some people like to write or dictate letters for young children or distant relatives and friends.

In general, finding out your relative's wishes early on will help prevent later difficulties.

Financial assistance for the carer.

If your relative would otherwise be an inpatient, you may be able to apply for the Carer Payment. This is not means tested and does not affect entitlements to pensions or other benefits and is not currently regarded as taxable income. Payment cannot be made for any period prior to your application being received.

A Carer Allowance is also available but certain conditions apply, such as the person in care receiving a DSS or Veteran Affairs Pension. Contact your nearest Centerlink office for up to date information.

The Cancer Council of Victoria has a Welfare Grant Fund. A diagnosis of cancer is needed to obtain assistance with day-to-day living expenses, but does not include medical and funeral expenses. Contact them or the equivalent organisation in your State or Territory.

What happens at the time of death?

You should know the physical changes that occur at this time and realise that mostly they do not require treatment, professional assistance or hospitalisation. It is simply the final act of living.

- As death approaches, people tend to become sleepier, sometimes confused, sometimes restless, difficult to rouse, not taking much food or drink. Vision may decrease.
- Secretions may collect at the back of the throat causing a 'rattle', which sounds more distressing than it really is, to the patient anyway.
- Urine output decreases and sometimes close to death, there may be loss of control of bladder and/or bowels.
- As circulation slows down color fades, the arms, legs, and finally the nose becomes cool to touch.
- Breathing is often more rapid initially, then irregular with seemingly long periods where no breathing occurs, until it finally ceases altogether.

What should you do?

- Talk calmly and be reassuring. Hearing is the last sense to be lost and your loved one may well be aware of your presence even if it is not acknowledged.
- Mouth swabs will relieve feelings of thirst, but don't attempt to make them swallow food or drink.
- Avoid excessive attempts to warm them up. Too many bedclothes or an electric blanket may make them restless.
- Incontinence pads and sheets will protect the patient and bedding.
- Elevating the head of the bed with pillows and turning the patient from side to side may relieve breathing problems.

- If the patient does seem to be distressed for any reason, the doctor or nurse may be able to help. Most times however, just being there, sitting with the patient and holding their hand is the most important thing to do.

How to tell if death has occurred.

There will be no breathing, no pulse, the eyes will be fixed in one spot with the pupils bigger than usual, and the mouth might be slightly open with the jaw relaxed.

What to do.

There is no hurry to do anything. Say your good-byes in your own time. If your relation dies through the night, it is all right to wait until the next day to notify the doctor and nurse, or it can be done straight away, the choice is yours. If there is going to be a delay, straighten the body after death before stiffness sets in.

Sooner or later a doctor must come to certify that death has occurred. The nurse may be able to help you wash your relative and dress them before you contact the funeral director. They will come and remove the body and guide you through the rest of the funeral arrangements. Before the funeral, you will have the opportunity to see your relation again if you wish.

Getting through the bereavement period.

Even though the death of your relative means the end of their physical suffering, it is still a sad event and can cause the greatest emotional pain you have ever experienced.

Everybody involved will need time and support to deal with feelings that may arise. Tears are the greatest release and healing, and contain a natural sedative.

Allow people to help you, particularly someone who

is willing to listen as you express your thoughts and emotions without judging or feeling the need to give advice. If you have difficulty or lack the opportunity to speak to someone, write down your feelings.

Don't neglect eating and sleeping and avoid taking inappropriate medication and excess alcohol. If possible, delay any big decisions.

Be aware that one of the ways to peace of mind is through forgiveness, of yourself and others. Let go of angry, judging or guilty thoughts, perhaps deciding it is more important to be happy than be justified as being right.

Grief counselling, support groups, books and articles on the grief process can provide support and reassurance, helping you survive the pain of your loss. Your palliative care volunteer if you have one, can be invaluable at this time.

There is no 'golden rule' on how long your grief will last, though three months seems to be an average time to come to terms with the reality and acute feelings. With someone to whom you were very close, there will always be an empty space in your heart and a longing to be with them again. I believe that if you just think of the one who has gone, their spirit will be with you and comfort you. Knowing you have done all you possibly could for them right up to the end should give you comfort and reason to be proud.

Appendix 6

Facts and Figures about Ovarian Cancer

Today, two more women in Australia died of ovarian cancer.

Around 75% of women with ovarian cancer (ovca) are already in advanced stage of the disease at diagnosis. Of these, some 80% will be dead within five years, many much sooner.

Frightening statistics for those diagnosed with this disease, but luckily it is rarer than other cancers. Young women in their teens, early twenties and older have been known to contract the disease, but it is most common over the age of forty, with the average age of diagnosis sixty-two years.

The lack of an effective screening test has lead to late diagnosis and, consequently, a high death rate. The five year survival rates are – Stage 1 - 90%, Stage 4 - 18%

My aim is to bring ovarian cancer to prominent public awareness, to educate women of the possible warning signs, and to encourage them to pursue diagnosis.

I have used the OVCA Australia website: **www.ovca.org**. But to source information, many women who are at risk do not have access to the Internet. This book is an avenue to pass on this vital information, and I am hoping that all who read it will pass it on to others.

Another useful website is that of the Cancer Council of Victoria: **www.accv.org.au**.

Remember, most women do not get ovarian cancer.

One in seventy women develop ovarian cancer, compared to one in seven or eight who will develop breast cancer. However, the ratio of deaths to new cases of ovca is an alarming 71%, whereas for breast cancer it is only 27%. The problem with ovca is that the symptoms can be very vague or even non-existent, so early detection is difficult. If it is caught in the early stages however, survival chances are 80 - 90%.

Risk factors.

Every woman is at some risk of ovca, regardless of age, heritage or medical history, but the following factors may increase your lifetime risk of developing the disease:

- You have two or more close relatives (like a mother, sister, or aunt) who have had ovca.
- You have a family history of multiple cancers: ovarian, breast, or colon cancer.
- You have a personal medical history of breast, endometrial (uterus), or colon cancer.

Other factors.

- You have a personal medical history of multiple exposures to fertility drugs.
- You are of Ashkenazi Jewish descent.
- You have had genital contact with talcum or asbestos, which are sometimes used in douches and condoms (highly controversial and unproven)

If you are at increased risk, ensure your doctor knows of the relevant medical family history.

There is some evidence that suggests that women who have not had children may be at a higher risk, although taking the contraceptive pill may significantly reduce the overall risk.

Early Symptoms.

While the symptoms of ovca, particularly in the early stages, are often not acute or intense, they are not always silent if you know what to look for, but may be vague and caused by other conditions. Medical research has shown that early-stage symptoms often exist. Take persistent signs seriously.

- Pelvic or abdominal pain or discomfort, and/or feeling of fullness.
- Bloating/swelling in the abdomen, unexplained weight gain; you look like you are suddenly pregnant.
- Weight loss; appetite loss.
- Feeling tired.
- Vague but persistent gastrointestinal upsets such as gas, nausea and indigestion.
- Backache.
- Cramps.
- Bladder or other urinary problems (frequency and/ or urgency of urination in absence of infection).
- Unexplained changes in bowel habits.
- 'Hard-feeling' ovaries.
- Unusual vaginal bleeding.
- Pain during intercourse.

Because many of the symptoms of ovca are similar to those of menopause, other gynecological conditions, or gastro-intestinal problems, tragic delays in diagnosis are quite common. If any of the symptoms appear, and they persist for more than a week or so, or if there is any reason to suspect you may have ovca, persist in getting a satisfactory explanation of your symptoms from your doctor and ensure that he or she has considered the possibility of ovca. If there is any doubt in your mind, be referred to the correct specialist, a gynecologic oncologist.

Ask to have the following important tests to help rule out ovarian cancer FIRST. (If there is no suspicion of ovca, then you can be tested for less deadly conditions)

- A recto-vaginal bimanual pelvic examination.
- A CA-125 or CEA (inhibin) blood test.
- A transvaginal ultrasound.

An experienced gynaecologist should perform the recto-vaginal bimanual pelvic examination.

If the results show an elevated CA-125 level and a mass in the pelvic area, see a gynaecologic oncologist, a surgeon who specializes in cancer of the reproductive system.

The best way to find ovarian cancer early.

If you are 18-40 years of age, having a recto-vaginal bimanual pelvic examination every 1-3 years while having your regular Pap smear would be a good idea. (Note: a Pap test can detect cervical, not ovarian cancer.) If you are over 40, a yearly check up as above is advisable. Women at risk would be wise to ask their doctor's advice on the frequency of checks.

If these examinations and the other tests mentioned show that ovca could be present, and if you have not already done so, you must see a gynaecologic oncologist.

In the experience and research of OVCA Australia Ltd, Melbourne, Australia, only those specialized in treating ovarian cancer are able to diagnose or dismiss it with any degree of accuracy.

The doctor will use your medical history and certain tests to learn more. Imaging tests like x-rays, computerized tomography (CT or CAT) scans, magnetic imaging (MRI) and ultrasound can show a picture of a tumor.

Australian Certified Gynaecologic Oncologists.

The membership of the Australian Society of Gynaecologic

Oncologists website at **http://www.users.bigpond.com/asgo** consists of gynaecologists certified by the Royal Australian College of Obstetricians and Gynaecologists as gynaecologic oncologists. Check that site for up-to-date listings of Australian Gynaecologic Oncologists.

Assess your risk.

At the website of the (USA) Women's Cancer Network, there is a confidential online form compiled by gynaecology cancer experts, which if completed, can assess the risk of developing breast, ovarian, endometrial and cervical cancer. No contact details need to be given except email to receive back the assessment. Do yourself a favor; take ten minutes of your time, complete the form, and get peace of mind; then pass this web site address on to every woman you know!

http://www.wcn.org/ Then click on the 'Risk' link.

If only I had had all this invaluable information at my fingertips in 1996, my story could have been very different.

Appendix 7

Hope for the future – latest research

Genetic testing for ovarian cancer

What is genetic testing?

The body contains millions and millions of cells. Within the cells is a nucleus, which contains the chromosomes. In each cell there are 46 chromosomes, which occur as 23 pairs. Genes are housed on the chromosomes. Genes are like the blue print of the physical body and they give messages to the cells of the body. The genes influence the body's growth, development and function.

Medical scientists are conducting huge amounts of research on the connection between human genes and health disorders. In some cases, the research has found a clear link between a particular gene mutation (an altered gene) and an inheritable disease. Members of a family where the disease occurs may then be able to be tested for the presence of the mutated gene to help them understand their risk of acquiring the disease.

For the purpose of this discussion, genetic testing falls into three broad categories.

1. Genetic tests that identify alteration(s) in genes for specific diseases that are known to be caused by a single dominant gene or a single pair of recessive genes. Such information enables prediction, with a high degree of certainty, whether an individual will

develop that particular disease. Each individual with a positive genetic test result will, however, not know precisely when the symptoms will onset or what the extent of the symptoms will be. Examples of specific diseases where such tests are readily available include Huntington's disease and Duchenne muscular dystrophy.

2. Genetic tests that determine a general predisposition to a certain disease or group of diseases. The risk may be due to an inherited mutated single gene or determined by the information contained in a number of different genes. Lifestyle and environmental factors need to be taken into account as these can increase or decrease the probability of a predicted disease occurring. Well-known examples of the influence of lifestyle and environment on the development of disease are smoking and lung cancer or sun exposure and skin cancer.
3. Genes that influence the course of various diseases that are not hereditary in nature. An example would be an analysis of any gene identified that influences the progression of HIV to AIDS.

Ovarian cancer fits into the second category.

Genetic testing specific to ovarian cancer

Two breast/ovarian cancer predisposition genes have been identified so far. They are called BRCA1 and BRCA2. Everybody has a pair of BRCA1 and BRCA2 genes and the normal message these genes give to the body is to keep check on cell growth and therefore prevent a cancer occurring. Cancer is a condition that occurs when there is uncontrolled cell growth. When there is a fault in a breast/ovarian cancer predisposition gene, the message the gene gives to the cell may be faulty and therefore there is an increased risk for cancer to develop. There are many steps involved in a cell changing from normal to cancerous. This is why having a fault in a breast predisposition gene (BRCA1 or BRCA2) increases the likelihood of cancer development but does not mean cancer will necessarily occur.

Genes always occur in pairs, as we inherit one of the pair from our mother and the other from our father. A person who has a fault in a breast/ovarian cancer predisposition gene has a pair of genes, one of which has a fault in it and the other which does not. Each time a child of that person is conceived, it is not possible to pass on both genes, as their partner also has to pass one on. Therefore there is a 50/50 chance of passing the faulty gene onto each child. Men and women can equally pass on these faulty breast/ovarian cancer predisposition genes, although rarely do men have health problems from such genes.

It is possible to test for faults in both BRCA1 and BRCA2 genes in some families. For this type of genetic testing it is necessary to obtain a blood sample from someone who has developed cancer. It is a time consuming process to find a faulty gene in an infected person, even in a high-risk family where the likelihood of finding a faulty gene is greatest. If a gene fault is identified, it means other family members could have a test to determine whether or not they have inherited the gene. The decision to have genetic testing is an individual one and best made after thinking through the advantages and disadvantages.

It is possible the genetic testing will not find a gene fault in BRCA1 or BRCA2. The explanation for this is that current technology for testing picks up most but not all faults, therefore, it is possible there is a gene fault but it has not been detected. There is also the possibility of yet another unknown gene in your family that causes an inherited predisposition to cancer. If the testing comes back and does not show a gene fault, it would still be suspected that your family might have a breast/ovarian predisposition gene.

The process of genetic testing

Adjacent to the Peter MacCallum Cancer Institute in Melbourne is the Jack Brockhoff Foundation Familial Cancer Centre. It is a clinic that provides genetic counselling, medical advice and psychological support to individuals and their families who are concerned about their family's history of cancer. These concerns include:

- Is there a gene in the family that is causing cancer?
- Am I at increased risk to develop cancer because of my family history?
- What are the risks to my children?
- Can I have genetic testing?

Following referral from your GP or Specialist, the genetic counsellor will telephone you to discuss your concerns and to collect information from you about the members of your family that have had cancer. There are certain features that are looked for in a family, which suggest there may be one of the cancer predisposition genes present. These include:

- Many close relatives on the same side of the family who have had breast/ovarian cancer.
- Family members who had breast/ovarian cancer diagnosed at a young age (30's and 40's).
- If you or a family member had a separate breast cancer in both breasts.
- The presence of other associated cancers, in particular ovarian cancer, in your family.

This information will help determine if your family has an increased risk of developing cancer. Gathering the necessary information may take several months, but it is important that as much detail as possible is obtained to provide you with an accurate assessment.

If your family is assessed as having an increased risk of developing cancer, you will be offered an appointment at the Familial Cancer Centre.

The first visit may take up to two hours and will involve a discussion with a genetic counsellor and medical specialist. They will ask about your concerns and review your family history. They will also provide you with information about the meaning of your family history, genes, cancer and genetic testing.

A second visit will be conducted a few weeks later to discuss issues regarding health surveillance, genetic testing, and its implications. You are asked to speak openly about your values, beliefs and personal health issues, and you are invited to bring your partner or friend for support if you wish.

This is a free service, so take your Medicare card and referral with you. All information you give is strictly confidential and the FCC will not directly contact other members of your family.

If it is decided there is a significant risk factor in your family, a small quantity of your blood is taken through a syringe for DNA testing for mutation analysis. The result can take 6-12 months. If the family mutation is identified, it is possible to offer predictive genetic testing to other relatives. This is a simpler procedure than mutation analysis, as the exact location of the mutation is known. This test usually takes less than four weeks, and gives a definite answer as to whether the person carries the family mutation.

When genetic test results become available, a genetic counsellor will call to arrange an appointment. The genetic counsellor and medical specialist meet prior to a results appointment to reflect on concerns the person may have.

The counsellor will take a couple of minutes to summarise the situation before giving the results as it may have been several months since the last visit to the clinic. Over 70% of mutation analysis testing conducted through the FCC comes back with an inconclusive result. This may result in a feeling of relief, frustration or disappointment.

Contact with the FCC does not finish with the result session. The counsellor will ring several weeks after an appointment to see how you have been feeling since receiving results. As the information received is often complex, a letter summarising the appointment is sent to help with understanding and recall. Further appointments are arranged as necessary.

Doctors treat genetic test results with the same care as any other medical information about you. This information is kept confidential as part of patient/doctor privilege. The doctor who ordered the test will not release the results unless you give written authority to do so.

Insurance

If and when you apply for life insurance, the insurance company may ask you to complete an application form and medical questionnaire. The medical questionnaire asks for details about your personal medical history, as well as information about any disease or disorders that are likely to increase the probability of a claim. It also asks basic questions about your medical history as this can indicate whether you may be at an increased risk of developing a hereditary disease.

The insurance company takes into account all the information on your application form and medical questionnaire to assess your likelihood of making a claim.

Unlike car or house insurance, once a life insurance policy has been issued, the insurance company cannot cancel or increase the price because of deterioration in your health. Insurance companies only get one chance to fully assess the risk; that is why so much emphasis is placed on assessing your risk at the beginning of the policy.

When a policy has been issued, subsequent changes in your health or the fact that you had a genetic test that was not previously contemplated will not impact on the price you pay for your existing insurance policy.

The search for early, accurate diagnosis

Researchers at the Peter MacCallum Cancer Institute in Melbourne are using a technique called mass spectrometry to look at blood samples to identify a 'fingerprint' (genomix). Their aim is to find a gene marker for ovarian cancer.

They are looking at as many blood samples as possible from women with ovarian cancer, and comparing them to women with benign ovarian disease. They are looking for a marker that is present in one and not the other.

CA-125 is an example of the kind of marker they are looking for. The problem with CA-125 is that it is often raised in benign disease and not always in ovarian cancers, particularly not early ones.

It is a huge fishing expedition that will take time.

New treatments

HMFG1

Trials are taking place at the Peter MacCallum Cancer Institute in Melbourne which involve the 'labelling' of cancer targeted antibodies with radioactive agents which aim to bind to cancer cells and release the radiation directly onto the cancer cells.

The agent is injected directly into the peritoneal cavity where most ovarian cancer recurrences occur.

The Austin Hospital in Heidelberg is also starting a new trial in this area of research.

OvaRex

This is a trade name for an antibody, an immune product, which targets abnormal cells through the body's immune system to CA-125 itself, and thus will target the body's immunity to CA-125.

The injection behaves like a vaccine, and in early studies on mice, has shown improved survival after this vaccination. It was then used in women with ovarian cancer to try and detect recurrence of disease by imaging (such as CT and PET scanning), and these women also showed improved survival.

This treatment has a low toxicity and could be a useful addition in the treatment of recurrent ovarian cancers.

It is currently in trials in the US, but not in Australia as yet.

Phenoxodiol

A pharmaceutical company in the US is presently trialling phenoxodiol on a number of cancers including recurrent ovarian cancer.

This particular chemical has been selected for its ability to inhibit two key targets on cancer cells that are critical to the growth and survival of most forms of cancer.

Within several hours of exposure to phenoxodiol, cancer cells display signs of distress. They stop dividing immediately, and die within 24-48 hours.

Phenoxodiol deprives the cancer cells of vital signals

that it needs to produce in order to continue to survive, thus allowing the body's immune system to kill the cancer cell.

The effect of phenoxodiol is limited to cancer cells and has no discernable adverse effect on non-cancer cells.

Phenoxodiol is administered orally in early-stage cancers where the treatment course is longer and by intravenous dosage for patients with late-stage cancer where the treatment course is of limited duration.

In some cancers, phenoxodiol appears to be strong enough to work on its own. However, one of its major benefits is its ability to condition cancer cells to the toxic effects of standard anti-cancer drugs. This is particularly helpful in ovarian cancer, which has become resistant to standard chemotherapies.

The drug is in Australia but is currently being trialled on prostate cancer.

For more information visit **www.phenoxodiol.com**

To keep track of current updates on known ovarian cancer research, visit **www.ovca.org**

REFERENCES

Appendix 1. **www.ovariancanada.org**

Appendix 2. **www.ovariancanada.org**

A Patients Guide to Radiation Therapy at the Peter MacCallum Cancer Institute

Appendix 3. **www.gyncancer.com/what-is.htm**

Appendix 4. **www.gyncancer.com/ovarian-cancer.html**

Appendix 5. *About Palliative Care*, issued by Palliative Care Victoria

Home Care by Eric Fairbank, Director of Palliative Care, Warrnambool & District Base Hospital

Appendix 6. **www.ovca.org/links**

Appendix 7. The Jack Brockhoff Foundation Familial Centre, Peter MacCallum Cancer Institute, East Melbourne, 2002/3

Investment & Financial Services Association LTD, March 2002

Bibliography

Bays, Brandon. *The Journey,* Harper Collins 1999

Chopra, Depac. *Quantum Healing; Ageless Body, Timeless Mind; Journey into Healing, The Path to Love,* Harmony Books 1997

Cilento, Ruth. *Heal Cancer*, Hill of Content 1993

Cotter, Arlene.*From This Moment On*, Pub. unknown

Clinkard, David. *The Uses of Juices*, Penguin 1992

Drum, David. *Making the Chemotherapy Decision,* Contemporary Books

Gawler, Ian. *You Can Conquer Cancer,* Hill of Content 1984

King, Petrea. *Quest for Life; Sometimes Hearts Have To Break,* Random House 1997

Lee, John R. *What Your Doctor May Not Tell You About Menopause,* Warner Books 1996

Leshan, Lawrence. *Cancer as a Turning Point,* Gill & Macmillan Ltd 1990

Meares, Ainslie. *Relief Without Drugs; The Wealth Within,* Hill of Content 1978

Myss, Caroline. *Anatomy of the Spirit*, Bantam Books 1996

Norwood, Robin. *Why Me, Why This, Why Now,* Arrow Books 1994

Siegal, Bernie. *Love Peace and Healing; Love Medicine and Miracles,* Harper Collins 1991

Thondup, Tulka. *The Healing Power of Mind,* Penguin Books 1996

Redfield, James. *The Celestine Prophecy,* Bantam Books 1995;

The Tenth Insight, Transworld 1997

Rinpoche, Sogyal, *The Tibetan Book of Living and Dying,* Vintage/Ebury 2002

Walsch, Neale, *Conversations With God Books 1,2 3; Friendship With God; Communion With God,* Hodder & Stoughton 1996 - 2000

New Releases...Also from Sid Harta Publishers

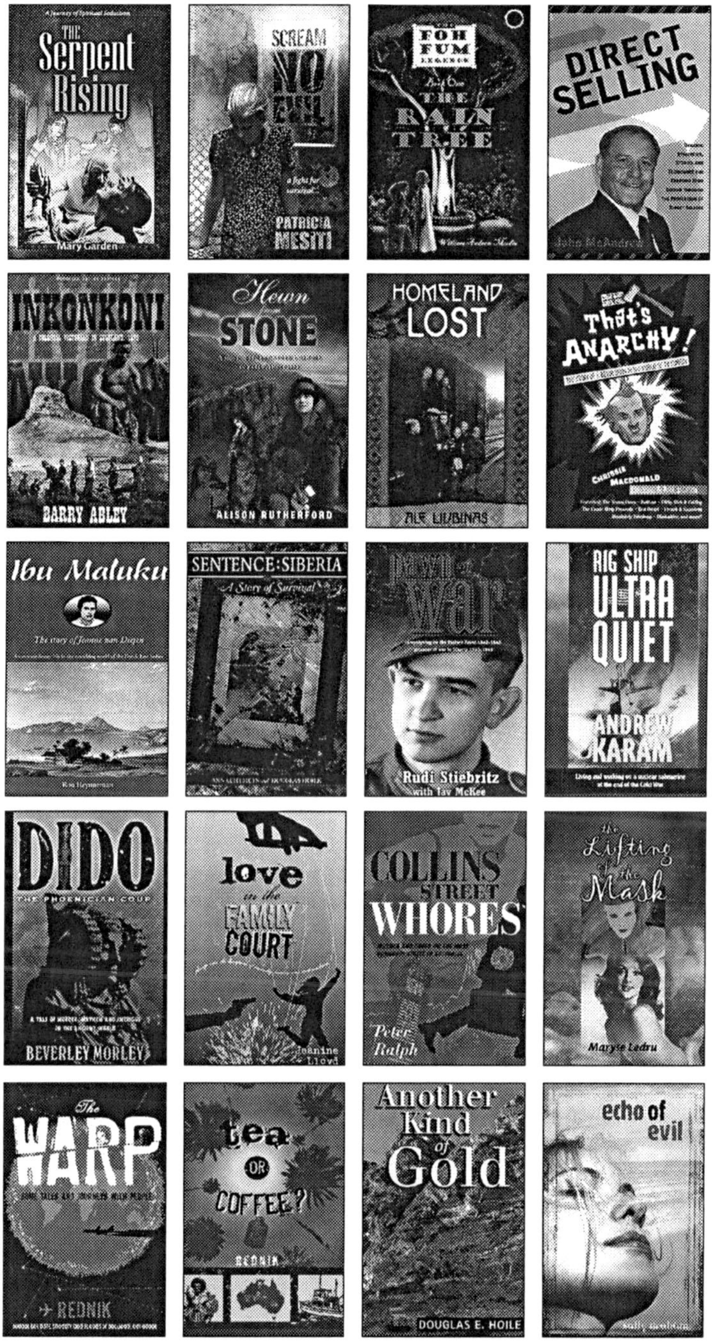

More New Releases

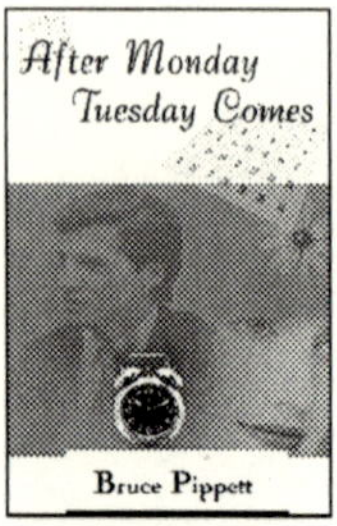

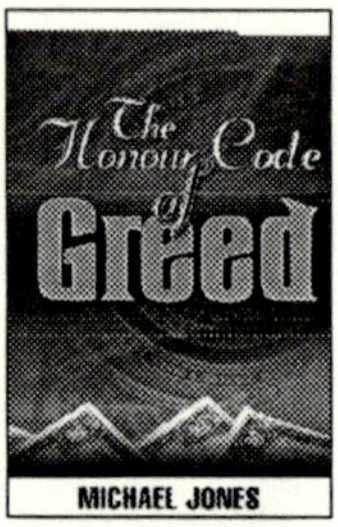

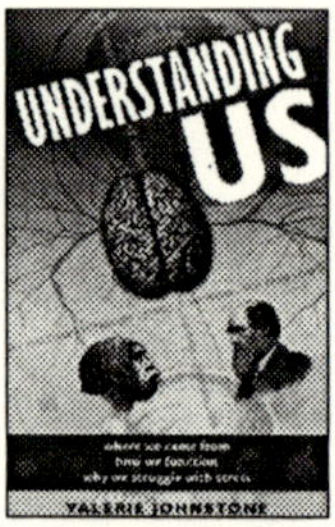

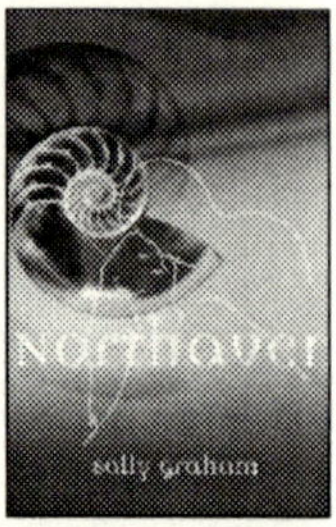

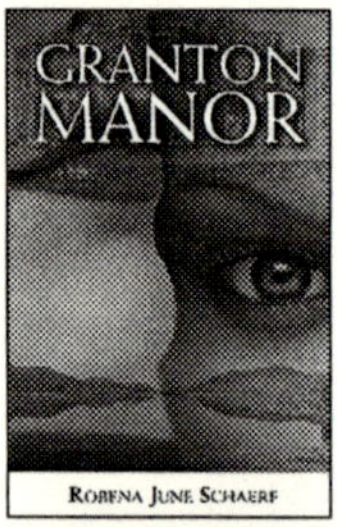

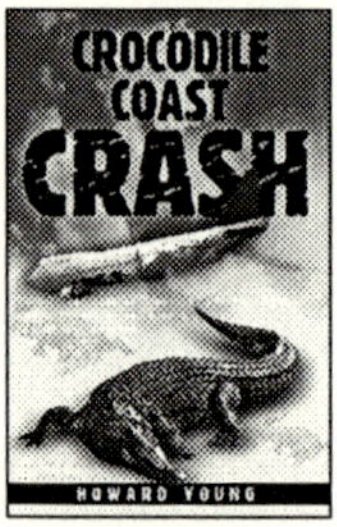

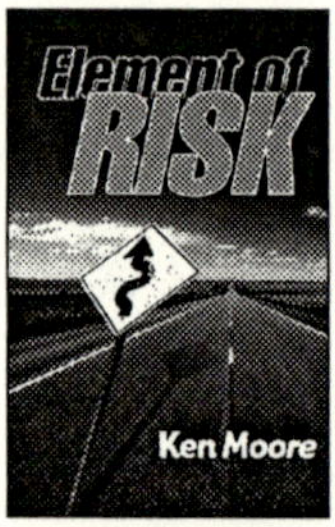

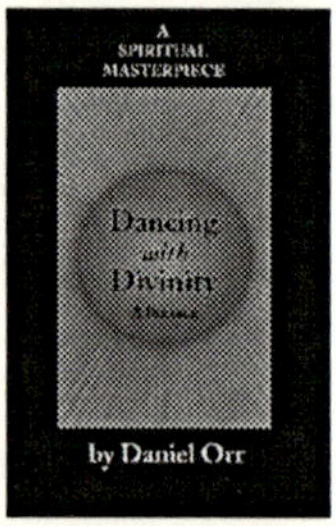

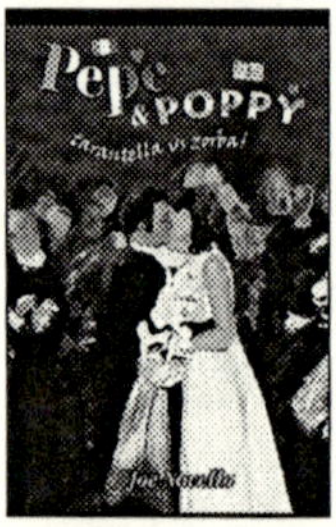

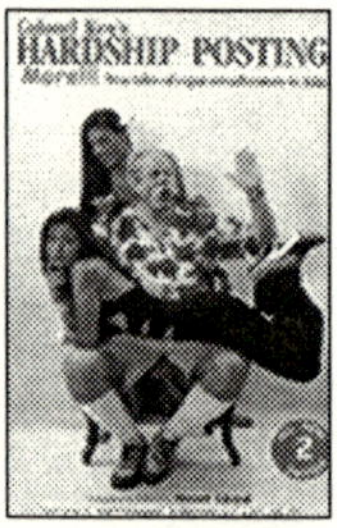

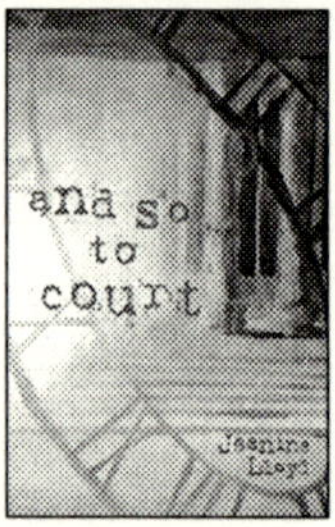

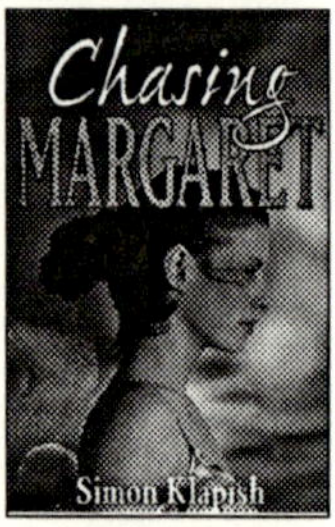

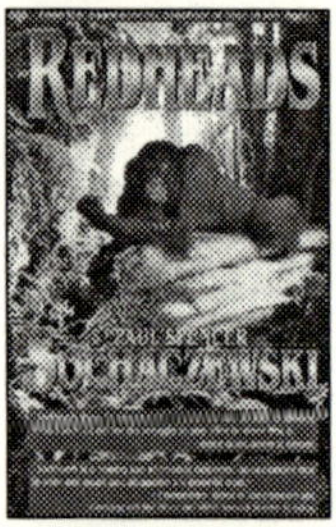

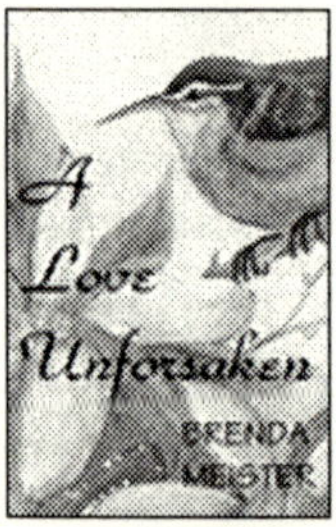

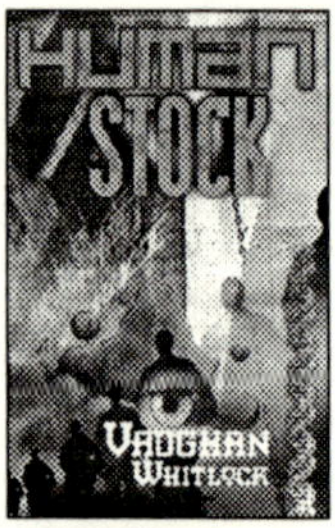

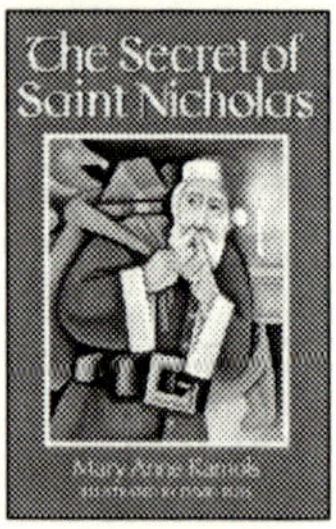

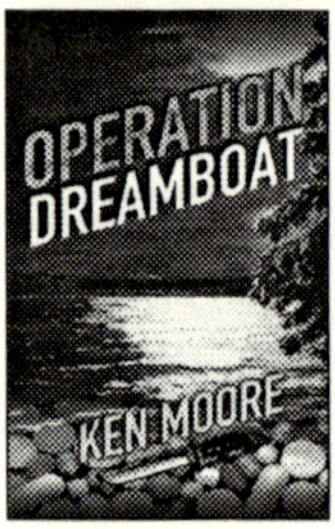

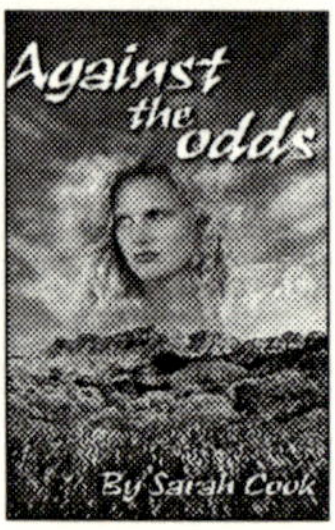

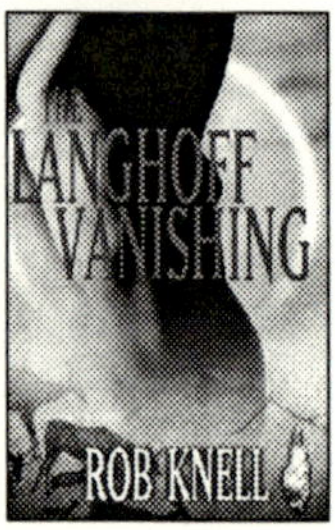

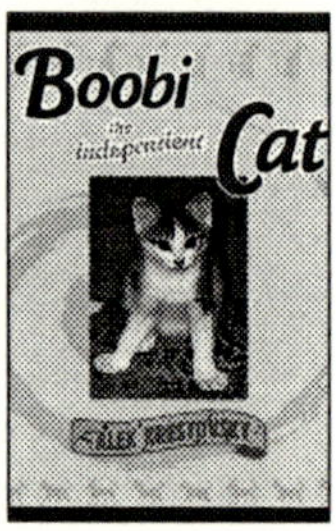

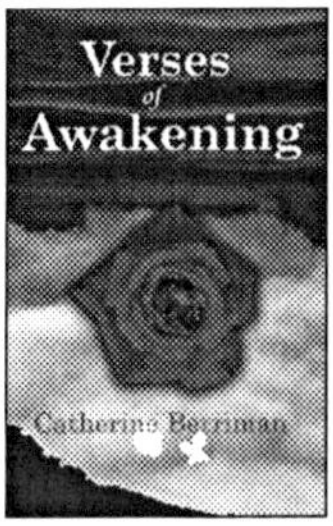

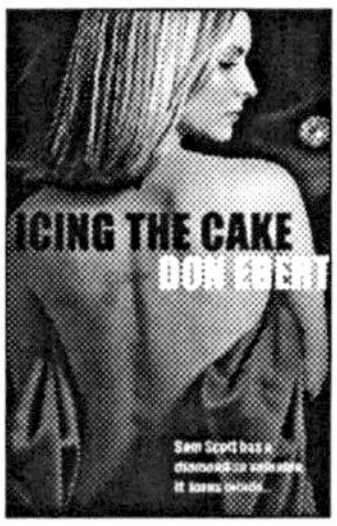

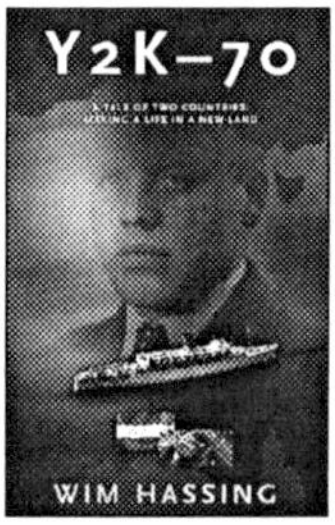

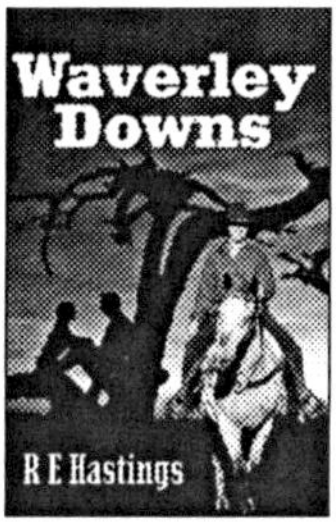

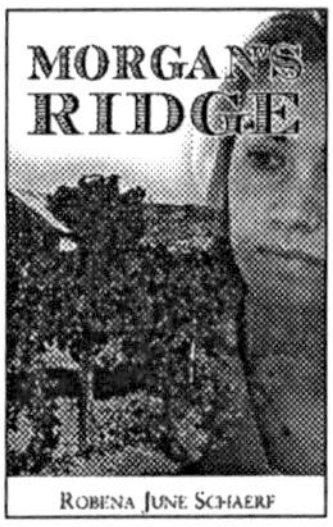

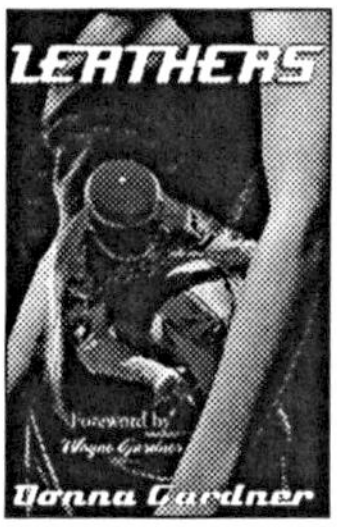

Best-selling titles by Kerry B. Collison

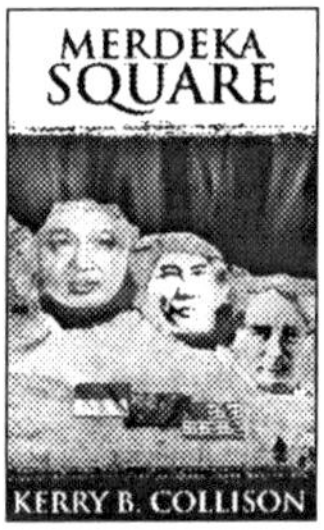

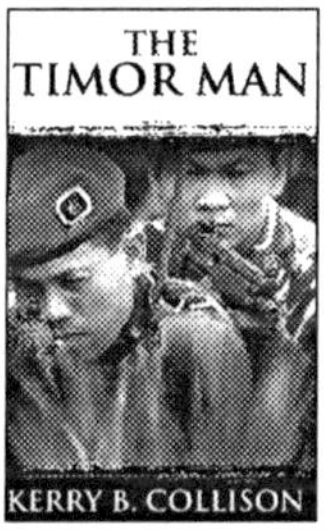

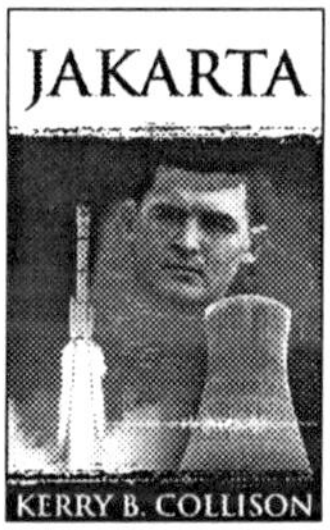

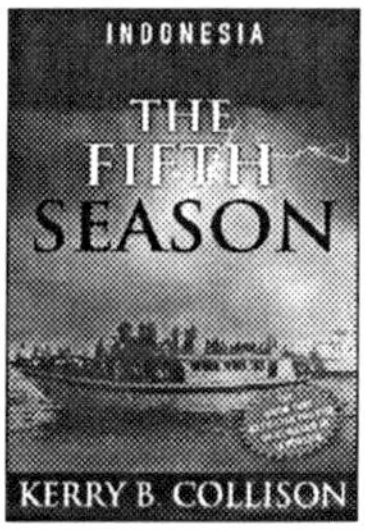

SID
HARTA
PUBLISHERS

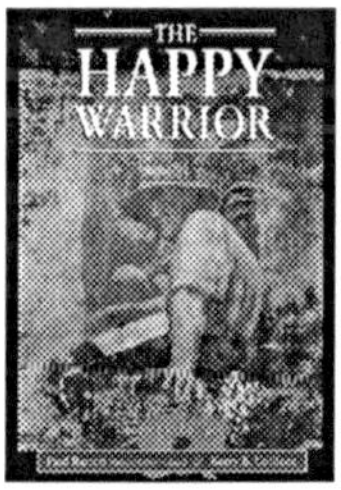

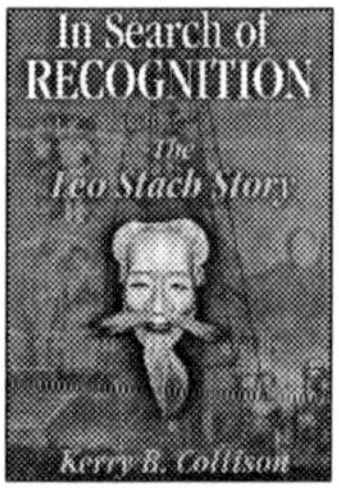

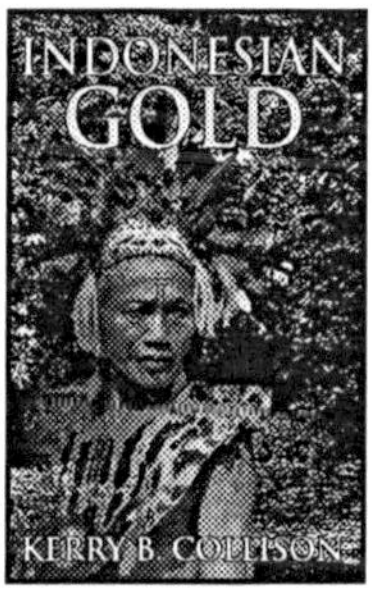

Printed in the United States
74584LV00002B/169

9 781877 059643